THE BIG
Dairy Free
COOKBOOK

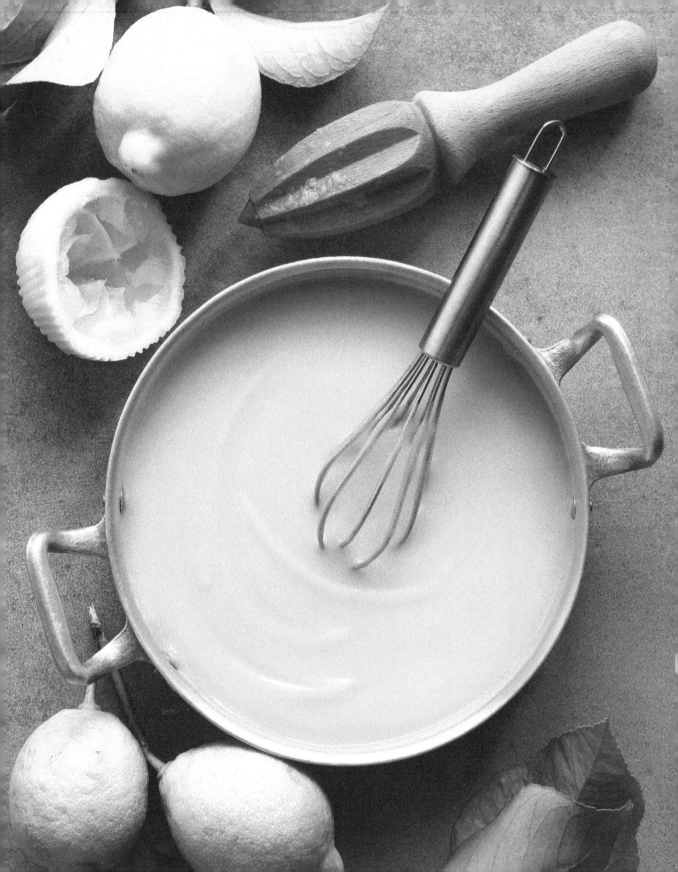

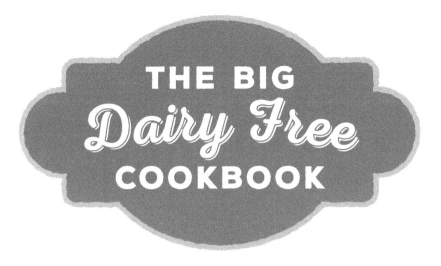

THE BIG Dairy Free COOKBOOK

THE COMPLETE COLLECTION OF DAIRY FREE RECIPES

Pamela Ellgen

ROCKRIDGE
PRESS

For general information on our other products and services or to obtain technical support, please contact our Customer Care Department within the United States at (866) 744-2665, or outside the United States at (510) 253-0500.

Rockridge Press publishes its books in a variety of electronic and print formats. Some content that appears in print may not be available in electronic books, and vice versa.

TRADEMARKS: Rockridge Press and the Rockridge Press logo are trademarks or registered trademarks of Callisto Media Inc. and/or its affiliates, in the United States and other countries, and may not be used without written permission. All other trademarks are the property of their respective owners. Rockridge Press is not associated with any product or vendor mentioned in this book.

Interior and cover design by Shubhani Sarkar

Photography © B. & E. Dudzinski/Stockfood, cover; The Picture Pantry/Stockfood, p. ii; Jennifer Davick, p. vi; Gräfe & Unzer Verlag/Coco Lang/Stockfood, p. 2; Trent Lanz/Stocksy, p. 10; Brigitte Sporrer/Stockfood, p. 18; Lisa Rees/Stockfood, p. 30; Magdalena Hendey/Stockfood, p. 50; Gräfe & Unzer Verlag/Mathias Neubauer, p. 66; Jonathan Gregson/Stockfood, pp. 86 & 104; Michael Wissing/Stockfood, p. 126; Eising Studio - Food Photo & Video/Stockfood, p. 184; Marti Sans/Stocksy, p. 202. Author photo © Rick Ellgen.

ISBN: Print 978-1-939754-58-5 | eBook 978-1-939754-59-2

Cover Image: Pepperoni, Red Onion, and Cherry Tomato Pizza ,page 106. Title Page Image: Lemon Curd, page 181.

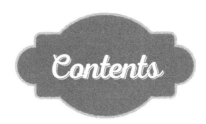

Contents

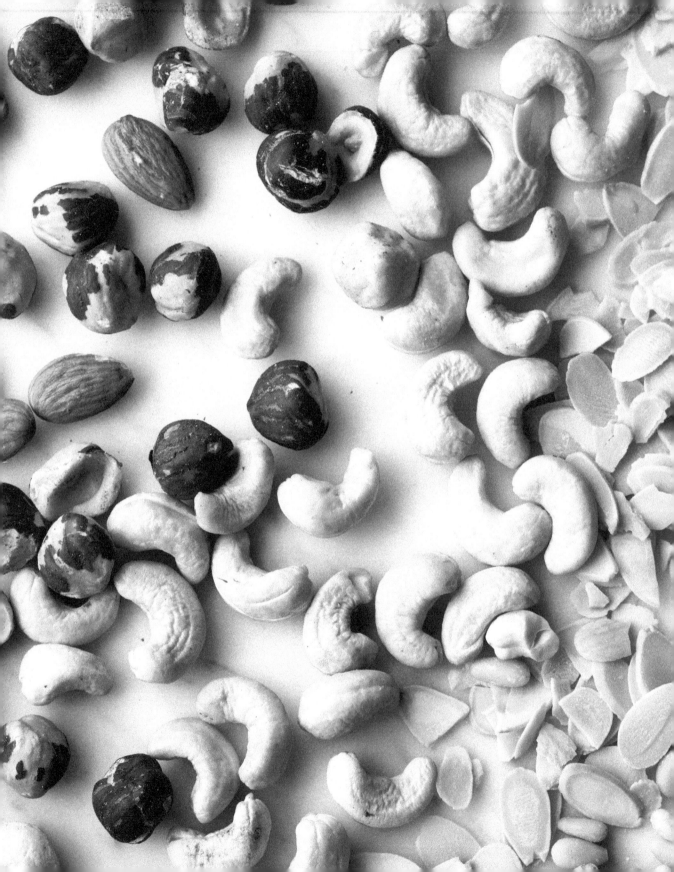

INTRODUCTION

One of my earliest memories is of speeding down the interstate in the front seat of my dad's Ford Thunderbird on the way to the hospital, hours after my bedtime. I tried to breathe, but every breath brought on wheezing and coughing that racked my seven-year-old body.

I was having an asthma attack triggered by dairy. It happened several times throughout my childhood and adolescence. I learned to live with it. I carried an inhaler and knew that especially after a cold, I was more susceptible to attacks. Even the thought of macaroni and cheese could leave me breathless.

As I grew older, I wanted to believe that I had outgrown the allergy. And, in some ways I had. The asthma attacks were mostly a thing of the past. So I indulged in pizza, ice cream, and plenty of artisan cheeses.

However, like so many adults, I eventually began to suspect that dairy might be the trouble behind numerous seemingly unrelated health concerns—gastrointestinal distress, mood changes, acne, and seasonal allergies. Whether these represented a true dairy allergy no longer mattered. When I cut dairy out of my diet for good, these issues all resolved themselves. The change was remarkable, and my newfound health made the sacrifice worth it.

Since then, I've found recipes that satisfy my cravings for nearly all my favorite foods. It's been a challenge. Some things can never be replaced—triple-cream Brie, for example. But my palate quickly changed to appreciate a dairy-free lifestyle—I even prefer to drink my coffee black now! And I've learned a lot along the way.

In this book, there's something for everyone. The easiest dairy-free route is to simply pick up store-bought analogues for dairy products—dairy-free cream cheese, dairy-free cheese shreds, etc. And in some instances, I do use those. But I prefer to diversify the ingredients, using white beans, nuts, and other naturally dairy-free ingredients to create creamy textures and divine flavors.

I'm excited to help bring new choices to your plate, and I hope that these recipes will help you feel great as you enjoy a dairy-free lifestyle that's satisfying, fun, and delicious!

Part One

HOW TO BE DAIRY FREE

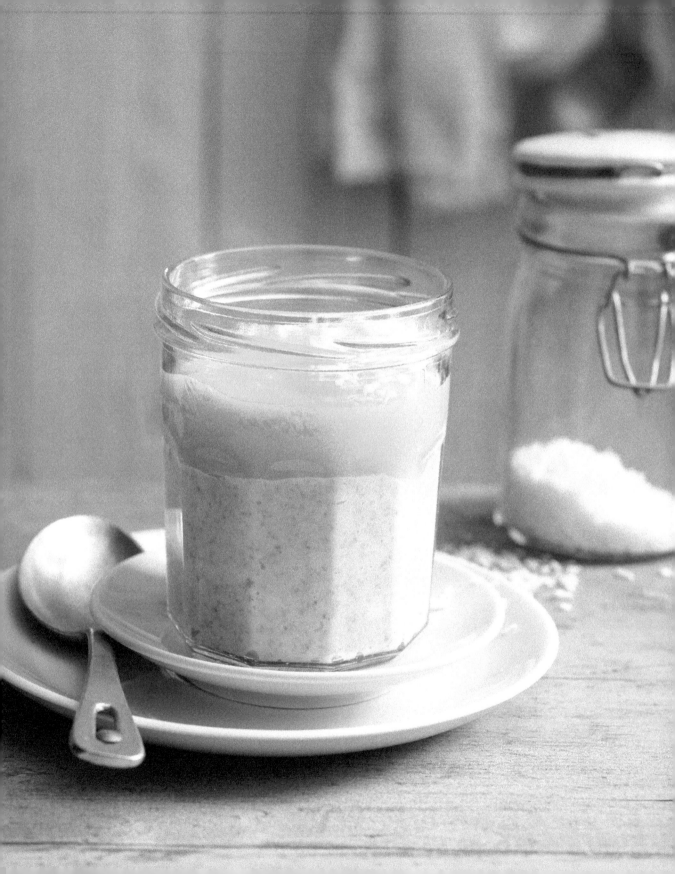

Chapter One

UNDERSTANDING THE DAIRY-FREE DIET

When you first embark on a dairy-free diet, it might seem as if dairy is in *everything*. Dairy products fill the pages of most cookbooks and sneak their way into ingredient lists of seemingly innocuous foods. The good news is, armed with a little bit of knowledge and the recipes in this cookbook, you can navigate the supermarket safely and smartly and create delicious meals you and your family will crave. This chapter will give you the basics to get started right away.

WHAT IS A DAIRY-FREE DIET?

Dairy products contain milk made from mammals—including cows, sheep, and goats—or from the by-products of milk production. Common dairy products include milk, cheese, butter, yogurt, cream, and ice cream. For the newly diagnosed, it may come as a relief to know that eggs are not dairy.

Some people restrict dairy from their diet for health reasons such as a milk allergy or lactose intolerance. Others avoid dairy for environmental or ethical concerns or religious reasons. Whatever your reason for giving up dairy, doing so can have a profound and positive impact on your health.

A strict dairy-free diet is essential for vegans or people with life-threatening allergies. This means that the obvious sources of dairy should be avoided, as well as all foods that contain a by-product of dairy, such as caseinates, whey protein, and hydrolysates (see Other Names for Dairy, page 6). Others choose to follow a generally dairy-free diet and avoid consuming obvious sources of dairy, but don't necessarily worry about foods that may contain a dairy by-product. This book follows a strict dairy-free diet.

DAIRY-FREE FOR BETTER HEALTH

You may be dealing with a new diagnosis that requires you to adopt a dairy-free diet, or perhaps you suspect that dairy may be the culprit behind chronic health issues. Let's look in some detail at the top health reasons to cut dairy from your diet.

Milk Allergy

Milk allergy is an immune reaction to milk that can involve hives, swelling, vomiting, wheezing, and potentially even anaphylaxis or death. A diagnosis is made by employing a food elimination diet, measuring antibodies in the blood, administering a skin-prick test, or some combination of these methods. The only proven treatment for a milk allergy is strict dairy avoidance. However, oral immunotherapy, which involves consuming miniscule but ever-increasing amounts of the allergen, has shown some promise in clinical settings.

A true milk allergy is relatively rare in adults, affecting only about 4 percent of the adult population. Conversely, it is the most common allergy among children. Additionally, because milk proteins can pass through breast milk to a breastfed baby, nursing mothers of children who are allergic to milk should also avoid consuming dairy products. Fortunately, the vast majority of children outgrow their milk allergy by the age of five.

Lactose Intolerance

Lactose intolerance is the inability to digest lactose, a sugar found in milk, because of an absence of the digestive enzyme lactase. This condition involves symptoms such as gas, bloating, nausea, and diarrhea, which occur when undigested lactose passes into the colon and feeds bacteria there. Lactose intolerance affects far more people than does milk allergy, perhaps as much as 65 percent of the global population. Individuals in Asia and central Africa are especially likely to be lactose-intolerant. One explanation for lactose intolerance is that before the advent of agriculture, human beings did not consume milk after weaning in early childhood, and their production of lactase ended. Lactase persistence, the body's manufacture of the lactase enzyme into adulthood, only began developing in European populations relatively recently, around 2000 BCE, and even more recently in cultures that did not rely on animal milk past weaning.

Food Sensitivity

Beyond lactose intolerance and true food allergies, which involve an immediate immune response, food sensitivities can cause reactions in people who are sensitive to dairy proteins. These reactions may include skin changes, mood disturbances, digestive problems, or other physical symptoms.

The best way to determine if you have a food sensitivity is to remove the suspected food for a period of 30 days, or until your symptoms subside, then reintroduce the food to see if a reaction occurs.

One explanation for food sensitivities is the "leaky gut" theory, which asserts that environmental and dietary factors have damaged the lining of the gut, creating spaces between the cells that line the intestinal tract. Larger protein molecules migrate from the digestive tract into the bloodstream, where the immune system mounts a response to the invaders. This may manifest in physical symptoms and potentially contribute to autoimmune disorders.

DAIRY SENSITIVITY CONNECTIONS

Individuals who have a dairy allergy are more likely to also be allergic to one of the other top eight allergens. In addition to dairy, these allergens are eggs, wheat, soy, fish, shellfish, peanuts, and tree nuts. US law requires these allergens to be listed on the label.

Unfortunately, proteins found in goat milk are similar to those in dairy and may also cause an allergic reaction. Interestingly, as many as 20 percent of children who are allergic to milk are also allergic to beef!

The recipes in this book are designed with these sensitivities in mind, and feature the "Allergen-Free" label for dishes that are free from all of the top eight allergens, or "Make Allergen-Free" for dishes that contain ingredients that can be easily swapped out to make them allergen-free.

Plant-Based Diet

A plant-based diet eliminates all animal products, including dairy, meat, eggs, fish, and poultry, and instead seeks all nutrition from plant sources. Numerous studies illustrate the health benefits of a plant-based diet, including reduced risks for heart disease, high blood pressure, type 2 diabetes, obesity, and other metabolic disorders; and conversely, improved gut microbiome diversity (a fascinating subject in itself), reduced cancer risk, and greater longevity.

Although they may look identical in practice, a plant-based diet is different from a vegan diet in that vegans avoid animal products in their lifestyle as well as in their diet, and do so for ethical reasons.

READING FOOD LABELS

Whatever your reasons for adopting a dairy-free diet, you'll want to know which foods contain dairy and which foods are at a high risk for cross-contamination. This section will help you decipher the sometimes-tricky food labels and screen for ingredients that contain dairy.

Be especially wary of foods labeled "non-dairy," a term used often on whipped cream, coffee creamer, and other processed foods, which legally can contain derivatives of dairy. Instead, seek out the label "dairy-free." How's that for confusing?

Dairy Foods

Here are the more obvious sources of dairy you probably already know to avoid.

- Butter
- Buttermilk
- Cheese
- Cottage cheese
- Cream
- Custard
- Ghee
- Half-and-half
- Milk
- Pudding
- Sour cream
- Yogurt

May Contain Dairy

These foods may contain dairy, but not always. Read the food label or ask the person who prepared it whether dairy is present.

- Artificial butter flavor
- Baked goods
- Caramel candies
- Chocolate
- Lunch meat, hot dogs, sausages
- Margarine
- Non-dairy products
- Nougat
- White/Alfredo sauce

GOOD NEWS— THAT'S NOT DAIRY!

After that lengthy list, it might feel as if dairy is lurking in everything! Fortunately, that isn't the case. In fact, several foods that sound suspiciously like dairy actually have nothing to do with milk products. These foods include eggs, shea butter, cocoa butter, malt vinegar, cream of tartar, and lactic acid.

Other Names for Dairy

Be on the lookout for these keywords that indicate the presence of dairy.

- Casein (a protein in milk)
- Casein hydrolysate
- Caseinates
- Diacetyl
- Lactalbumin
- Lactalbumin phosphate
- Lactoferrin
- Lactose (the main sugar in milk)
- Lactulose
- Milk protein hydrolysate
- Recaldent
- Rennet casein
- Sour milk solids
- Tagatose
- Whey (the watery part of milk)
- Whey protein hydrolysate

GETTING CALCIUM AND VITAMIN D

The first thing people—even random strangers—ask when they hear that you don't eat dairy is, "But how do you get your calcium?" The dairy industry has made it seem like an unquestionable fact that cow's milk is the ideal source of calcium for humans and consuming it is the only way to prevent osteoporosis.

However, a panel of scientists at the United States Department of Agriculture (USDA) came to another conclusion in 2001 when they investigated the claims made in the ubiquitous "milk mustache" ads. They found that there was no evidence that dairy consumption alone builds strong bones or prevents osteoporosis. The panel also found that whole milk consumption may contribute to heart disease and prostate cancer.

How Much Do You Need?

Undeniably, calcium and vitamin D are essential nutrients for human health. The Recommended Dietary Allowance (RDA) for calcium is 1,000 milligrams a day for men and women ages 19 to 50, increasing to 1,200 milligrams for women over 50 (for men, it remains at 1,000). The RDA for vitamin D is 600 IU (15 mcg) for men and women ages 19 to 70.

Calcium and vitamin D work in tandem—among other benefits, vitamin D increases calcium absorption in the gut and maintains calcium and phosphate balance to ensure normal bone mineralization.

Vitamin D and Calcium Sources

Rest assured, you will get your calcium. Calcium is available from a wide array of foods unrelated to dairy. In fact, some of these foods have additional health-promoting elements, including vitamins, minerals, antioxidants, and fiber. Foods that naturally contain calcium include sardines, broccoli, watercress, edamame, figs, almonds, beans, tofu, salmon, collard and turnip greens, kale, bok choy, and oranges. Some processed foods are also fortified with calcium, such as soy milk, orange juice, and even chocolate.

Few foods in nature contain vitamin D, according to the National Institutes of Health, and the only reason milk is seen as a good source of the vitamin is because it has been fortified. Other foods are also fortified, including breakfast cereals, orange juice, and other processed foods. Whole food options include swordfish, salmon, tuna, beef liver, and egg yolk.

The primary method our bodies enlist for obtaining adequate (80 to 90 percent) vitamin D is sun exposure to bare skin (sunscreen blocks out the rays that help your body manufacture the vitamin). The amount of time required for your skin to produce adequate vitamin D varies based on the time of year, your location, your skin color, and how much skin you have exposed (more is better). It's essential to note that adequate vitamin D production can occur in half the time that it takes for your skin to begin to burn.

Beyond getting adequate sunlight, other common-sense lifestyle factors can improve your vitamin and mineral stockpile, such as exercising, ceasing smoking, and limiting caffeinated beverages and sodas.

Supplements

Nutrition supplements may be helpful to ensure adequate levels of calcium and vitamin D, especially on a dairy-free diet. However, it's important to consult with your physician to have your nutritional status tested before you start taking pills.

Calcium supplements come in the form of calcium citrate, malate, and carbonate, with carbonate being the most common. It is the primary ingredient in TUMS, for example. However, it is the least absorbable and should be taken with food to be most effective. Some supplements offer a combination of calcium types. Supplements are best divided into multiple doses, because the body cannot absorb large amounts of calcium at one time.

Vitamin D supplements are an option for people living in extreme latitudes, those with darker skin, and older individuals. However, supplementation is a tricky thing; it can result in kidney stones, arterial calcification, and high concentrations of calcium in the blood— good reasons to talk with your doctor first.

DAIRY-FREE LIVING SUCCESS

After living strictly dairy-free for the past four years, I know the ins and outs of staying dairy-free, and I know I'm supposed to tell you that it's always been easy. But, at least initially, it can be challenging. You might be saying goodbye to some of your favorite foods, which are often tied to deeply personal experiences and cultural traditions. You may also be dealing with children who aren't thrilled that you're taking away their beloved dishes (and if so, I want to reassure you that there *is* a mac and cheese recipe in this book!).

You may be asking, what in the world *should* I eat? Here are my tips and tricks for going dairy-free with grace.

Handling Cravings

There are a few strategies that work for me when it comes to handling cravings. First, I go without. Yes, you read that right, but keep reading; I'll get to a solution. Most dairy-free substitutes on the market just don't cut it for me. There are some that do, but most just remind me of what I'm missing, and they aren't all that healthy. Instead of accepting an unsatisfactory substitute, I skip the cream in my coffee and mostly choose family grill night over pizza night.

Second, I invest a little more energy into preparing delicious foods that are naturally dairy-free. You'll definitely want to try my Coconut-Ginger Pork Tenderloin Skewers (page 109) or Sweet Potato Nachos with Barbecued Tempeh (page 148). In fact, most Asian cuisine across the board is naturally dairy-free and tastes amazing. When you look beyond the standard American diet, a world of naturally dairy-free cuisine awaits. By exploring the options, you're likely to develop a whole list of new foods to crave— and these you *can* enjoy!

Finally, as if going back on my first strategy, I sometimes splurge on dairy-free prepared foods when a craving for something creamy, salty, or sweet strikes. There are some good ones. Miyoko's Creamery products, Trader Joe's Soy Creamy Cherry Chocolate Chip ice cream, Earth Balance Buttery Spread, and Tofutti Better than Sour Cream are some of my favorites. I also have developed recipes for this book that offer some of the features of dairy that I missed most—the saltiness and creaminess, especially. I think my Miso-Tahini Ice Cream (page 173) is to die for, and Plant-Based Parmesan (page 27) is close enough to the real thing that it does the trick.

For some people, dairy cravings go beyond simply missing your favorite foods. In the book *The Cheese Trap*, Dr. Neal Barnard argues that dairy contains mild opiates that attach to the same brain receptors that heroin and morphine do, causing us to eat more than we should and keep coming back. Fortunately, when dairy is removed from the diet, eventually the cravings subside. For some people, this happens within a few days. For others, it can take as long as two weeks.

Dining Out

Some decisions are easy; you know to pass on the cheesy pizza and loaded nachos when dining out, but it's also important to be aware of hidden sources of dairy in restaurant cooking. Things you would never think contain dairy, such as roasted vegetables or pan-seared meat, are often topped with butter just before serving. Many baked goods contain dairy, as do mashed potatoes, pancakes, scrambled eggs, and other seemingly non-dairy foods.

I recommend calling restaurants ahead of time or checking their websites to learn about their dairy-free options. Vegan restaurants are an easy solution, but not if you're looking for meat. Restaurants serving Thai, Japanese, and Chinese cuisine are usually completely dairy-free. When you arrive, inform your server of your needs and ask him or her to point you to some dairy-free options on the menu, and request that the chef please skip the butter on your dish.

Eating at Social Gatherings

Dietary restrictions have become more commonplace, lessening the feeling of social stigma and making it easier to navigate social gatherings. It's good to inform your host of your dietary restrictions when you accept an invitation. I usually quickly follow this up with an offer to bring a side or main dish to share. If it's a small gathering, such as dinner at someone's house, I often suggest the many things I still do eat. Most hosts find this helpful, because they may have never even considered what foods do or don't contain dairy (and in my case, gluten). If I suspect that the situation may not provide sufficient dairy-free options, I'll eat a small protein-rich snack before I arrive.

Kids' Parties and School Celebrations

Birthday parties can be so hard for little ones who sit there watching their friends devour cupcakes, ice cream, and pizza. I don't want my children to feel deprived or socially awkward, so on these occasions, I tell the host about their dietary restrictions and offer to bring something they can eat. I try to match it as closely as possible to whatever else is being served. For birthday parties in the classroom, it's easiest for me to supply the teacher with a cache of individually wrapped treats that my kids can have whenever birthday parties pop up throughout the year. I also have tried keeping a stash of cupcakes in my freezer. I can easily defrost them one at a time and send them to school when I know another kid is celebrating a birthday.

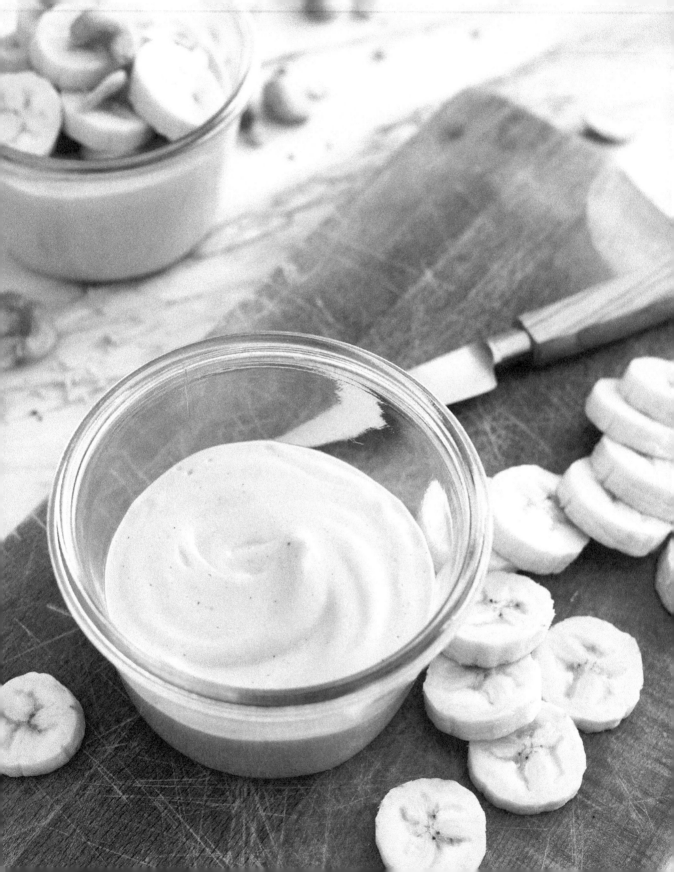

Chapter Two

THE JOY OF DAIRY-FREE COOKING

Dairy-free cooking has become more than a necessity in my kitchen—it has become fun! I love finding alternatives to dairy that taste delicious and keep my whole family healthy. There's something particularly satisfying about creating a new ice cream recipe or discovering a fabulous hot nacho cheese dip. Soon you, too will be having fun (yes, *fun*) cooking without dairy.

PREPARING YOUR KITCHEN

Naturally, a well-stocked pantry and refrigerator filled with dairy-free foods for meals and snacks makes cooking easy, especially when hunger strikes and you need food in a hurry. Shopping is actually more enjoyable than you might imagine. After I changed my diet, I gave myself permission to spend a little more than usual and try new foods I might have otherwise considered a splurge.

Preparing the kitchen also involves removing any items containing dairy, both the obvious sources and those hiding behind the sneaky dairy ingredients listed in chapter 1 (see page 6). Some couples and families in which only one person needs to be dairy-free might choose to leave dairy foods in the house. Others choose to go completely dairy-free. In my home, we usually opt for the latter. It's just not fair for one kid to get a loaded pizza and the other to get a dairy-free version while sitting at the same table. (We have tried several brands of dairy-free cheese, and my son Brad can always tell the difference.)

ESSENTIAL EQUIPMENT

Beyond the basics—pots, pans, knives, cutting boards, and utensils—a few kitchen appliances and gadgets will make dairy-free cooking easier, tastier, and more fun. Fortunately, there are only a few items that I consider essential to a dairy-free diet. These items are used primarily to make staples such as almond milk, which saves money, eliminates packaging waste, and avoids the thickeners and preservatives in store-bought varieties.

Blender: for making smoothies, plant-based milks, and sauces

Food processor: for chopping and grating vegetables, and grinding nuts

Ice cream maker: for preparing homemade dairy-free ice cream

Nut milk bag: a reusable muslin or nylon bag with a drawstring for straining plant-based milks and cheeses

MAKE YOUR OWN NUT MILK BAG

As the saying goes, desperation is the mother of invention, so if you find yourself without a nut milk bag, make your own. Spread a few layers of cheesecloth over a large metal strainer, and pour the nut milk mixture through it. Gather the corners of the cheesecloth and twist to squeeze out as much liquid as you can.

STOCKING A DAIRY-FREE PANTRY

Here are the most important basic ingredients to always have on hand for easy preparation of dairy-free meals, snacks, and drinks.

Almonds: for making almond milk

Cashews: for making cashew cream and using in sauces

Coconut milk: for making curries and soups, and using in place of cream when the flavor is complementary. Alternatively, homemade coconut milk can be made from shredded unsweetened coconut.

Dairy-free butter: to replace butter as a condiment and in cooking (but generally not in baking). I recommend Earth Balance Buttery Spread. If you have a soy allergy, make sure to purchase the soy-free version and use it when making recipes labeled "Make Allergen-Free" that call for this ingredient.

Dairy-free chocolate chips: for making cookies, trail mix, and other sweet treats

Dairy-free sour cream: for making sauces, thickening soups, and as a condiment

Non-hydrogenated vegetable shortening: for baking

Nutritional yeast: for giving sauces and dips a cheesy flavor. Available online and at health foods stores in bulk or prepackaged. (This is not a yeast for baking or brewing—it is not a leavener.)

Silken tofu: for thickening sauces and making desserts (different from soft or firm tofu)

HOW TO COOK WITHOUT DAIRY

You can approach dairy-free cooking in a few different ways. The first and easiest option is to choose naturally dairy-free

three approaches. I offer recipes
that never had dairy to begin with. I use
store-bought replacements for dairy in a few
recipes. And I offer many recipes that use
novel ingredients to stand in for dairy.

Common Substitutions

Butter: In cooking, I use canola oil instead
of butter. It has a higher smoke point, so
it doesn't burn, and it has a neutral flavor.
I also opt for olive oil or coconut oil if the
flavor is desirable in the recipe. In baking, I

use non-hydrogenated vegetable shortening
or coconut oil in place of butter. However,
since butter isn't pure fat and contains
some liquid, I add about 1 tablespoon of
plant-based milk or water for every cup of
butter that's called for.

Soft cheeses: For fresh soft cheeses such as
ricotta, queso fresco, and chèvre, I usually
opt for a nut-based cheese. I like the flavor
of macadamia nuts, cashews, and blanched
almonds best, and I add some lemon juice
or vinegar for acidity. Firm tofu can also
be pulsed in a food processor to take on the
consistency of ricotta.

Hard cheeses: I love my Plant-Based Parmesan
(page 27), which combines cashews, garlic
powder, salt, and nutritional yeast in a
crumbly, dairy-free triumph. It is not built
for slicing but is delicious sprinkled over
pasta, pizza, salad—okay, pretty much
everything!

Cheese sauce: For a sauce, I have found
several options that work, including silken
tofu, blended cashews, and white sauce
made with oil, starch, and plant-based milk.
White beans and other vegetables can also
be blended into a convincing sauce. Check
out my Mac 'n' Cheese (page 149) and
Creamy Artichoke and Pesto Pizza (page 147)
for two different cheese sauce options, in
addition to the cheesy dip and sauce
recipes in chapter 6, Snacks and Sides.

Cream: Full-fat coconut milk and Cashew
Cream (page 22) both work well as a substitute for cream in cooking and baking. When

THE JOY OF DAIRY-FREE COOKING

chilled, store-bought coconut milk can whip into soft, fluffy peaks like whipped cream.

Milk: Plant-based milks work well in most recipes calling for milk. I use my basic Plain Nut Milk (page 20) in most recipes calling for milk, and it fills the need. You can also use soy milk. Rice milk, however, has a thinner texture and should only be used when that consistency is desirable.

Yogurt: For cooking and baking, coconut milk with a splash of lemon juice stands in nicely for yogurt in many recipes. Store-bought dairy-free yogurts are hit or miss, with many containing nothing more than plant-based milk, thickener, probiotics, and loads of sugar. You can also make your own dairy-free yogurt, but it is more difficult to get right than homemade yogurt made with dairy.

PLANT-BASED MILKS

Plant-based milks are healthy substitutes for dairy milk, and they taste pretty good, too. Each non-dairy milk has a slightly different flavor, and they often vary greatly with regard to nutritional profiles. What they don't have is cholesterol, lactose, antibiotics, or hormones.

You can purchase all of the plant-based milks listed here at the grocery store, or make your own at home. This book offers a full chapter of such recipes. I like the convenience of purchasing plant-based milk, but I prefer to avoid the thickeners, stabilizers, emulsifiers, and other additives that often reside in store-bought milks. Plus, I just think the ones I make at home taste far better! The one exception is that for cooking, I prefer store-bought canned coconut milk and coconut cream.

The table on the next page offers nutrition facts for 1-cup servings of the most common plant-based milks. Note the two entries for coconut milk. The first is a coconut milk beverage, usually stored in the refrigerated section or in a shelf-stable carton. The second is for canned coconut milk used in cooking but not as a beverage by itself.

Almond milk: The most common nut-based milk, almond milk has a fairly neutral flavor and aroma. Depending on the ratio of almonds to water, almond milk can have a full body without the need for thickeners. It is easy to make at home and to find in stores.

Cashew milk: With a slightly stronger, nuttier flavor, cashew milk is excellent for cooking and making ice creams. It is easy to make at home, though it requires slightly more effort than almond milk to squeeze in a nut milk bag.

Coconut milk: This plant-based milk is sold as a beverage in cartons and in cans for use in cooking. It contains saturated fat, but it is considered healthy because the fat is in the form of lauric acid, a medium-chain fatty acid that is easily converted to usable energy. Despite its name, coconut contains no actual nuts, so it is typically safe for those with a nut allergy (but always consult your physician if you have a life-threatening allergy).

1-CUP SERVING	CALORIES	FAT	SATURATED FAT	PROTEIN	CARBOHYDRATES	FIBER
ALMOND MILK	30	2.5	0	1	1	1
CASHEW MILK	25	2	0	1	1	0
COCONUT MILK BEVERAGE	45	4	3.5	0	<1	0
COCONUT MILK, CANNED	420	42	36	3	9	0
MACADAMIA MILK	50	5	1	1	1	1
OAT MILK	130	2.5	0	4	24	2
QUINOA MILK	70	1	0	2	12	0
RICE MILK	70	2.5	0	0	11	0
SOY MILK	100	4	.5	8	8	1

Rice milk: Rice milk has a thinner body and more carbohydrates than other plant-based milks. It is another good alternative for those with a nut allergy.

Soy milk: This plant-based milk bears the most nutritional resemblance to dairy milk of all the plant-based milks, with 8 grams of protein per serving. It has a mild aftertaste, however, and many people who are allergic to dairy are also allergic to soy.

Part Two

RECIPES

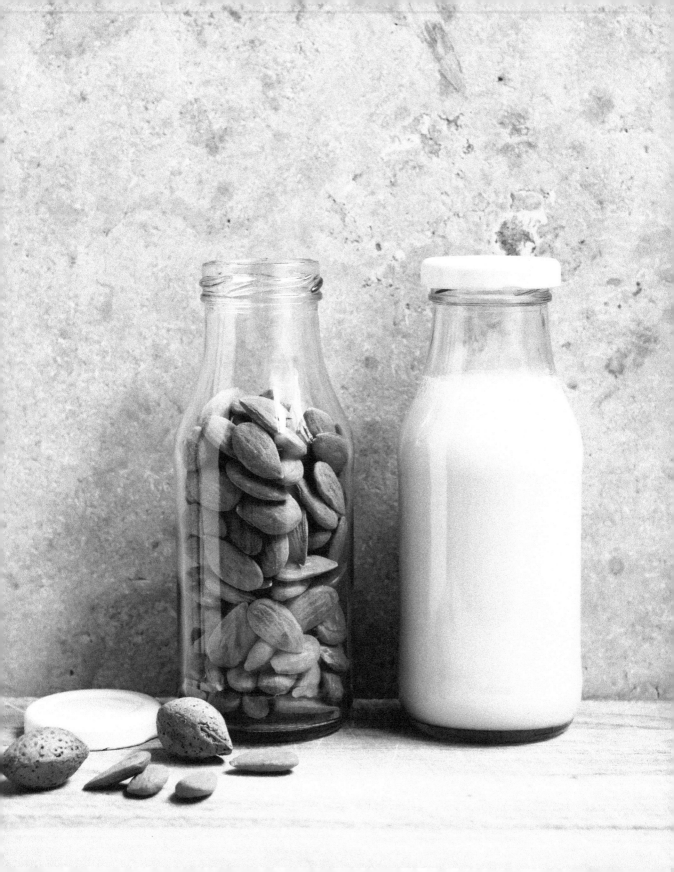

PLANT-BASED MILKS AND CHEESES

PLAIN NUT MILK

Egg-Free, Gluten-Free, Vegan

YIELD: 4 cups (32 ounces)

PREP TIME: 5 minutes

You can make this nut milk with a variety of nuts—try almonds, hazelnuts, cashews, or Brazil nuts. My go-to is almonds because the flavor is relatively neutral, and they're inexpensive. Plain nut milk is a great starting point, and it works better in savory cooking than sweetened vanilla nut milk, but you can take it in so many directions. Add strawberries or chocolate, or toast the nuts before blending.

1 cup raw nuts   Pinch sea salt

4 cups water, divided

Per Serving (1 cup) Calories: 37; Total Carbohydrates: 2g; Sugar: 0g; Total Fat: 3g; Saturated Fat: 0g; Sodium: 168mg; Protein: 1g; Fiber: 1g

1. In a blender, combine the nuts, 1 cup of water, and the salt. Purée until very smooth.

2. Add the remaining 3 cups of water, and blend for 30 seconds.

3. Pour the mixture through a nut milk bag, and squeeze the bag to extract all the liquid.

4. Store the nut milk in a covered container in the refrigerator for up to 5 days. It will separate slightly, but simply shake the container to homogenize.

INGREDIENT TIP: Make the nuts easier to blend and more digestible by soaking them in fresh water for 2 hours or up to overnight. Rinse them thoroughly and drain before proceeding with the recipe.

VANILLA NUT MILK

Egg-Free, Gluten-Free, Vegan

YIELD: 4 cups (32 ounces)

PREP TIME: 5 minutes

Vanilla Nut Milk is useful in baking, serving over cereal, blending into a smoothie, or just adding to your morning coffee. You can use maple syrup, pitted dates, or another sweetener of your choice in this recipe. I prefer the natural sweetness of dates.

1 cup raw nuts
(almonds, hazelnuts, cashews, or Brazil nuts)

2 pitted dates or 1 tablespoon maple syrup

1 teaspoon vanilla extract

4 cups water, divided

Pinch sea salt

Per Serving (1 cup) Calories: 53; Total Carbohydrates: 5g; Sugar: 3g; Total Fat: 3g; Saturated Fat: 0g; Sodium: 169mg; Protein: 1g; Fiber: 1g

1. In a blender, combine the nuts, dates, vanilla, 1 cup of water, and the salt. Purée until very smooth.

2. Add the remaining 3 cups of water, and blend for 30 seconds.

3. Pour the mixture through a nut milk bag, and squeeze the bag to extract all the liquid.

4. Store the nut milk in a covered container in the refrigerator for up to 5 days. It will separate slightly, but simply shake the container to homogenize.

INGREDIENT TIP: Use leftover nut milk pulp in place of almond flour in baked goods such as muffins, pancakes, or cookies. It has slightly more moisture and less fat than almond flour, but it works well in most recipes. If you're not ready to use it right away, it can be stored in a covered container in the refrigerator for up to 5 days.

CASHEW CREAM

Egg-Free, Gluten-Free, Vegan

YIELD: 1½ cups (12 ounces)

PREP TIME: 5 minutes, plus 30 minutes to soak

Cashews are my go-to nut for making a thick, velvety cream. You can use this cream to make sauces, dairy-free ice cream, and baked goods. However, unlike heavy cream, you cannot whip it into stiff peaks—for that, use chilled, store-bought coconut cream.

1 cup raw cashews   Pinch sea salt

1½ cups water, divided

Per Serving (2 tablespoons) Calories: 80; Total Carbohydrates: 4g; Sugar: 1g; Total Fat: 6g; Saturated Fat: 1g; Sodium: 0mg; Protein: 2g; Fiber: 1g

1. In a medium bowl, cover the nuts with boiling water and leave to soften for 30 minutes.

2. Rinse the nuts until the water runs clear.

3. In a blender, combine the nuts, 1 cup of water, and the salt. Purée until very smooth.

4. Add the remaining ½ cup of water, and blend for 30 seconds.

5. Pour the mixture through a nut milk bag, and squeeze the bag to extract all the cream.

6. Store the cream in a covered container in the refrigerator for up to 5 days. It will separate slightly, but simply shake the container to homogenize.

SERVING TIP: Blend this recipe with 1 cup of coconut milk, a splash of vanilla extract, and 1 tablespoon of maple syrup for a delicious coffee creamer.

SOY MILK

Egg-Free, Gluten-Free, Nut-Free, Vegan

YIELD: 4 cups (32 ounces)

PREP TIME: 5 minutes, plus 12 hours to soak

COOK TIME: 20 minutes

While it's not as easy to make as nut milk, soy milk is a good source of protein and is naturally nut-free. Soybeans (not to be confused with edamame, the young, green soybean) must be cooked to make them digestible, so make sure to heat the blended soybean mixture to at least 180° F and maintain this temperature for the full cooking time.

¾ cup yellow soybeans

4 cups water, divided, plus 4 cups water for soaking the soybeans

Pinch sea salt

Per Serving (1 cup) Calories: 80; Total Carbohydrates: 4g; Sugar: 1g; Total Fat: 4g; Saturated Fat: 1g; Sodium: 85mg; Protein: 7g; Fiber: 1g

1. In a medium bowl, cover the soybeans in 4 cups of water and leave to soak for at least 12 hours.

2. Rinse the soybeans until the water runs clear.

3. Remove the soybean skins as thoroughly as possible, then transfer the hulled soybeans to a blender. Add 2 cups of water and the salt.

4. Blend until mostly smooth. Add the remaining 2 cups of water, and continue to blend until very smooth.

5. Pour the mixture through a nut milk bag, and squeeze the bag to extract all the liquid.

6. Transfer the soy milk to a medium saucepan over medium heat and bring to a simmer. Simmer for 20 minutes, skimming foam off the surface as it rises.

7. Allow the soy milk to cool completely and then transfer to a covered container. Store in the refrigerator for up to 5 days.

COOKING TIP: To make a sweetened vanilla soy milk, simply add 1 teaspoon of vanilla extract and 2 pitted dates or 1 tablespoon of maple syrup with the soybeans in step 3.

COCONUT MILK

Egg-Free, Gluten-Free, Nut-Free, Vegan

YIELD: **4 cups (32 ounces)**

PREP TIME: **5 minutes**

This coconut milk makes a fantastic dairy-free ice cream and can be used in cooking or enjoyed as a delicious beverage. Unlike the canned coconut milk found in the grocery store, this version is thinner and does not contain any gums or emulsifiers.

1 cup shredded unsweetened coconut flakes

4 cups water, divided

Pinch sea salt

Per Serving (1 cup) Calories: 45; Total Carbohydrates: 1g; Sugar: 1g; Total Fat: 4g; Saturated Fat: 4g; Sodium: 35mg; Protein: 0g; Fiber: 0g

1. In a blender, combine the coconut, 1 cup of water, and the salt. Purée until very smooth.

2. Add the remaining 3 cups of water, and blend for at least 30 seconds.

3. Pour the mixture through a nut milk bag, and squeeze the bag to extract all the liquid.

4. Store the coconut milk in a covered container in the refrigerator for up to 5 days. It will separate slightly, but simply shake the container to homogenize.

VARIATION TIP: To make a flavorful toasted coconut milk, toast the coconut in a large dry skillet until gently browned, about 5 minutes, then follow the recipe as directed.

RICE MILK

Allergen-Free, Egg-Free, Gluten-Free, Nut-Free, Vegan

YIELD: 4 cups (32 ounces)

PREP TIME: 5 minutes

Once you realize how ridiculously easy it is to make homemade rice milk, you'll know exactly what to do with that leftover Chinese takeout container of rice—milk it! You can use either white or brown rice in this recipe. Because most of the rice grain is left behind, there is little difference between white and brown in the amount of fiber extracted.

1 cup cooked rice

4 cups water, divided

Pinch sea salt

Per Serving (1 cup) Calories: 65; Total Carbohydrates: 11g; Sugar: 1g; Total Fat: 2g; Saturated Fat: 0g; Sodium: 110mg; Protein: 0g; Fiber: 0g

1. In a blender, combine the rice, 1 cup of water, and the salt. Purée until very smooth.

2. Add the remaining 3 cups of water, and blend for 30 seconds.

3. Pour the mixture through a nut milk bag, and squeeze the bag to extract all the liquid.

4. Store the rice milk in a covered container in the refrigerator for up to 5 days. It will separate slightly, but simply shake the container to homogenize.

SERVING TIP: Transform this milk into a delicious Mexican horchata by adding ½ teaspoon of ground cinnamon, ½ teaspoon vanilla extract, and 2 tablespoons brown sugar or maple syrup.

QUINOA MILK

Allergen-Free, Egg-Free, Gluten-Free, Nut-Free, Vegan

YIELD: 4 cups (32 ounces)
PREP TIME: 5 minutes

Quinoa is considered a pseudo-grain, meaning it is usually served like a grain but is actually a seed. It is an excellent source of protein and makes a strongly flavored milk. It is especially good when blended into smoothies or used as a liquid in baking for an added boost of protein.

1 cup cooked quinoa   Pinch sea salt

4 cups water, divided

Per Serving (1 cup) Calories: 70; Total Carbohydrates: 12g; Sugar: 2g; Total Fat: 1g; Saturated Fat: 0g; Sodium: 0mg; Protein: 2g; Fiber: 0g

1. In a blender, combine the quinoa, 1 cup of water, and the salt. Purée until very smooth.

2. Add the remaining 3 cups of water, and blend for 30 seconds.

3. Pour the mixture through a nut milk bag, and squeeze the bag to extract all the liquid.

4. Store the quinoa milk in a covered container in the refrigerator for up to 5 days. It will separate slightly, but simply shake the container to homogenize.

INGREDIENT TIP: If you have leftover quinoa but don't want to make quinoa milk right away, you can store it in a resealable bag in the freezer for up to 3 months until ready to use. Allow it to thaw for about 10 minutes before blending.

PLANT-BASED PARMESAN

Egg-Free, Gluten-Free, Vegan

YIELD: 1 cup

PREP TIME: 5 minutes

I know it's culinary sacrilege, but I once actually liked those green cans of Parmesan. There was something about the dry, salty bits showered over pizza or pasta that just worked for me. Fortunately, the dairy-free version of canned Parmesan is easier to replicate than aged Parmesan wedges.

1 cup unsalted raw cashews

¼ cup nutritional yeast

1 teaspoon sea salt

1 teaspoon garlic powder

Per Serving (2 tablespoons) Calories: 109; Total Carbohydrates: 8g; Sugar: 0g; Total Fat: 6g; Saturated Fat: 1g; Sodium: 234mg; Protein: 7g; Fiber: 3g

1. Combine all the ingredients in a small food processor, and pulse until finely ground.

2. Transfer the mixture to a covered container, and store at room temperature indefinitely.

   COOKING TIP: When blending the Parmesan, a clean coffee grinder does a nice job. To avoid overcrowding the machine, blend it in batches.

BASIC NUT CHEESE

Egg-Free, Gluten-Free, Vegan

YIELD: 1¼ cups

PREP TIME: 5 minutes, plus 30 minutes to soak

You can make this nut cheese with blanched almonds, cashews, or macadamia nuts. It works beautifully in dairy-free lasagna, crêpes, or other recipes where ricotta cheese is called for. It's especially important to soak the nuts before blending, otherwise you'll need to add too much water to get the blender going.

1 cup raw nuts

¼ cup water, plus more if necessary, plus 2 cups boiling water for soaking the nuts

2 tablespoons freshly squeezed lemon juice

¾ teaspoon sea salt

Per Serving (¼ cup) Calories: 126; Total Carbohydrates: 6g; Sugar: 0g; Total Fat: 10g; Saturated Fat: 2g; Sodium: 73mg; Protein: 4g; Fiber: 1g

1. In a medium bowl, cover the nuts with 2 cups of boiling water and leave to soak for 30 minutes. Alternatively, cover them with cold water and soak overnight.

2. Rinse the nuts until the water runs clear.

3. In a blender, combine the nuts, ¼ cup of water, the lemon juice, and salt. Purée until mostly smooth, adding up to another ¼ cup of water if necessary.

4. Store the nut cheese in a covered container in the refrigerator for up to 5 days. It will separate slightly, but simply shake the container to homogenize.

SERVING TIP: To make a scrumptious spreadable cheese, stir in 1 tablespoon of minced shallots and 1 tablespoon of minced fresh herbs such as rosemary, tarragon, or basil.

TOFU RICOTTA

Egg-Free, Gluten-Free, Nut-Free, Vegan

YIELD: 2 cups

PREP TIME: 10 minutes

I use the Basic Nut Cheese (page 28) and this tofu ricotta interchangeably when making Lasagna (page 150). This version is lighter in texture than regular ricotta but has a great flavor. Also, don't be tempted to skip the sugar in this recipe; milk contains naturally occurring sugars, so adding sugar to the tofu is essential to recreate a similar flavor.

14 ounces firm tofu, drained and broken into pieces

¼ cup extra-virgin olive oil

2½ tablespoons freshly squeezed lemon juice

2 teaspoons sugar

1 teaspoon minced garlic

1 teaspoon sea salt

Per Serving (¼ cup) Calories: 94; Total Carbohydrates: 2g; Sugar: 1g; Total Fat: 8g; Saturated Fat: 1g; Sodium: 241mg; Protein: 4g; Fiber: 1g

1. In a food processor, combine all the ingredients.

2. Blend until mostly smooth.

   VARIATION TIP: To make a sweet tofu ricotta, omit the garlic and reduce the salt to ½ teaspoon.

   INGREDIENT TIP: The quality of tofu you use really does matter here. I use Wildwood Organic Sprouted Tofu.

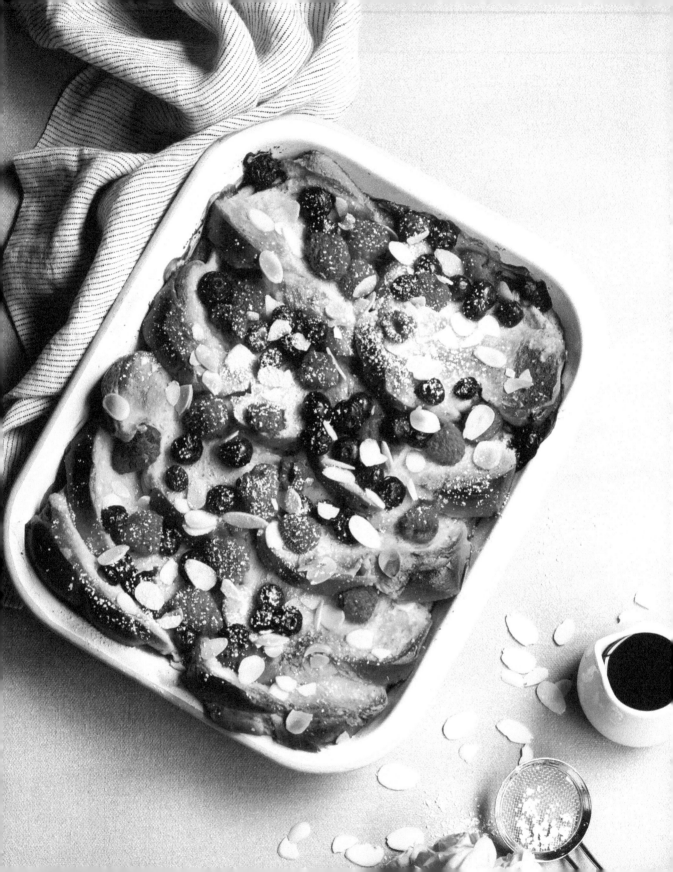

Chapter Four

SMOOTHIES AND BREAKFAST

French Toast, page 38

CREAMY BANANA-ALMOND PROTEIN SHAKE

Egg-Free, Gluten-Free, Make Allergen-Free, Make Nut-Free, Vegan

SERVES 1

PREP TIME: 5 minutes

This is my favorite breakfast. I drink it nearly every single day, especially on busy mornings when I want to sneak in a workout before rushing the kids off to school and heading to work. It's cool, creamy, and packed with plant-based protein. I highly recommend freezing the diced banana ahead of time for especially thick and creamy results.

1 medium banana, diced, frozen

1 cup Vanilla Nut Milk (page 21) or store-bought unsweetened almond milk

½ to 1 cup ice

1 serving chocolate dairy-free protein powder (see Ingredient tip)

Per Serving Calories: 285; Total Carbohydrates: 41g; Sugar: 16g; Total Fat: 7g; Saturated Fat: 1g; Sodium: 311mg; Protein: 16g; Fiber: 11g

1. In a blender, combine the banana, nut milk, and ½ cup of ice. Pulse until mostly smooth, adding more ice as desired.

2. Add the protein powder and blend until smooth, scraping down the sides with a spatula as needed.

INGREDIENT TIP: My favorite plant-based protein powders are the sport versions of Vega and Garden of Life in chocolate flavor. These are sweetened with stevia, contain 30 grams of protein per serving, and don't contain soy.

SUBSTITUTION TIP: To make this allergen-free, use Rice Milk (page 25) or Quinoa Milk (page 26) instead of the Vanilla Nut Milk.

GREEN MONSTER SMOOTHIE

Allergen-Free, Egg-Free, Gluten-Free, Nut-Free, Vegan

SERVES 1

PREP TIME: 10 minutes

I introduced this to my boys at an early age, and they quickly slurped it down. It's a convenient way to serve them dark leafy greens while they're still a little suspicious of salads. To make this a complete meal, serve with a handful of nuts or a healthy protein bar.

¼ to ½ cup water

1 cup firmly packed kale or spinach

1 lime, peeled

1 small banana, peeled

½ cup frozen diced pineapple

Small handful fresh cilantro (optional)

Small handful fresh parsley (optional)

Per Serving Calories: 199; Total Carbohydrates: 52g; Sugar: 24g; Total Fat: 1g; Saturated Fat: 0g; Sodium: 33mg; Protein: 4g; Fiber: 7g

In a blender, combine all the desired ingredients. Purée until very smooth, adding just enough water to blend.

INGREDIENT TIP: To peel the lime, cut off each end with a sharp knife, and then stand it on one end and slice away the outer peel.

CHERRY PIE SMOOTHIE

Egg-Free, Gluten-Free, Make Allergen-Free, Make Nut-Free, Vegan

SERVES 1

PREP TIME: 5 minutes

This smoothie features the creamy texture and sweet, tart flavor of a cherry pie with ice cream. I add vanilla protein powder for a boost of flavor and nutrition, but it is optional, especially if you're making it for a snack instead of a meal.

1 cup Vanilla Nut Milk (page 21) or store-bought unsweetened vanilla almond milk, or allergen-free plant-based milk

1 small banana, diced, frozen

½ cup frozen cherries

1 serving vanilla dairy-free protein powder (optional)

Per Serving Calories: 341; Total Carbohydrates: 52g; Sugar: 27g; Total Fat: 9g; Saturated Fat: 1g; Sodium: 422mg; Protein: 23g; Fiber: 11g

1. In a blender, combine the nut milk, banana, and cherries, and pulse until mostly smooth.

2. Add the protein powder (if using) and blend until smooth, scraping down the sides with a spatula as needed.

SERVING TIP: This smoothie is even more decadent with a handful of dairy-free dark chocolate chips stirred in.

PIÑA COLADA SMOOTHIE

Allergen-Free, Egg-Free, Gluten-Free, Nut-Free, Vegan

SERVES 1

PREP TIME: 5 minutes

Close your eyes and let this tropical treat deliver you to a faraway place. This virgin breakfast smoothie is filled with healthy fats from the coconut milk and complex carbs. For added nutrition, include a scoop of vanilla protein powder.

1 cup Coconut Milk (page 24)

Juice of ½ a lime

1 small banana, diced, frozen

1 cup frozen diced pineapple

Per Serving Calories: 238; Total Carbohydrates: 53g; Sugar: 31g; Total Fat: 5g; Saturated Fat: 4g; Sodium: 4mg; Protein: 2g; Fiber: 7g

In a blender, combine all the ingredients, and purée until smooth.

VARIATION TIP: If you want to turn this into a grown-up drink, who am I to stop you? Add 3 ounces of white rum and divide the smoothie into two portions.

APPLE PIE OATMEAL

Egg-Free, Gluten-Free, Make Allergen-Free, Make Nut-Free, Vegan

SERVES 4

PREP TIME: 5 minutes   COOK TIME: 5 minutes

My kids adore hot cereal for breakfast, especially this quick and easy apple pie oatmeal with all the flavors of the classic dessert. This dish takes just a few minutes longer than the instant oatmeal packets to prepare, but contains a fraction of the sugar.

2 cups old-fashioned oats

2 apples, peeled, cored, and diced

1 teaspoon ground cinnamon

1 teaspoon vanilla extract

¼ teaspoon sea salt

4½ cups water

4 teaspoons brown sugar

4 teaspoons dairy-free butter, such as Earth Balance Buttery Spread

¼ cup finely chopped pecans, optional

¼ cup Vanilla Nut Milk (page 21)

Per Serving Calories: 158; Total Carbohydrates: 23g; Sugar: 7g; Total Fat: 7g; Saturated Fat: 1g; Sodium: 167mg; Protein: 3g; Fiber: 3g

1. In a large saucepan over medium heat, stir together the oats, apples, cinnamon, vanilla, salt, and water, bringing it to a simmer.

2. Cover, reduce the heat to low, and simmer for 5 minutes.

3. Divide the oatmeal between four serving bowls, and, one by one, top with the sugar, dairy-free butter, pecans (if using), and nut milk.

SUBSTITUTION TIP: To make this allergen-free, use soy-free dairy-free butter, omit the pecans, and use a nut- and soy-free milk.

CREAMY OATMEAL WITH CARAMELIZED BANANAS

Egg-Free, Gluten-Free, Make Allergen-Free, Make Nut-Free, Vegan

SERVES 4

PREP TIME: 5 minutes   COOK TIME: 10 minutes

If your morning oatmeal has become a predictable routine, change it up with this recipe for a real treat! This creamy, decadent breakfast borders on dessert and is a good fit for the weekend. But the caramelized bananas are a cinch to make, so you can really serve it any day of the week.

2 cups old-fashioned rolled oats

2 cups Coconut Milk (page 24)

2 cups Plain Nut Milk (page 20) made with almonds

¼ teaspoon sea salt

1 tablespoon vanilla extract

1 tablespoon coconut oil or canola oil

2 medium bananas, cut into ½-inch-thick slices

1 tablespoon brown sugar

4 teaspoons dairy-free butter, such as Earth Balance Buttery Spread

¼ cup finely chopped toasted hazelnuts

Per Serving Calories: 364; Total Carbohydrates: 29g; Sugar: 8g; Total Fat: 26g; Saturated Fat: 10g; Sodium: 463mg; Protein: 4g; Fiber: 5g

1. In a large saucepan over medium heat, stir together the oats, coconut milk, almond milk, salt, and vanilla, bringing it to a simmer.

2. Cover, reduce the heat to low, and simmer for 5 minutes.

3. While the oatmeal cooks, in a large skillet over medium-high heat, heat the oil.

4. Sprinkle the banana slices on both sides with the sugar. Arrange them in a single layer in the skillet, and cook for about 2 minutes, until nicely caramelized but not blackened. Flip carefully, and cook for another 2 minutes.

5. To serve, divide the cooked oatmeal between four serving bowls, top with the caramelized bananas, and then top with the dairy-free butter and hazelnuts.

SUBSTITUTION TIP: To make this nut-free and allergen-free, substitute the almond milk with coconut milk and omit the hazelnuts.

INGREDIENT TIP: If you're short on time and want to ditch some of the fat and sugar in this recipe, skip caramelizing the bananas and just serve raw banana slices on the oatmeal. It's still delicious!

FRENCH TOAST

Make Gluten-Free, Make Nut-Free, Vegetarian

SERVES 4

PREP TIME: 5 minutes COOK TIME: 25 to 30 minutes

French toast, a timeless decadence, is easily made dairy-free using Vanilla Nut Milk, but you can try it with any plant-based milk in this recipe. If you opt for an unsweetened milk, add a splash of vanilla extract and maple syrup to the batter.

1 tablespoon oil

2 eggs

1 cup Vanilla Nut Milk (page 21)

½ teaspoon ground cinnamon

2 tablespoons coconut oil or canola oil, divided

10 slices wheat bread or gluten-free bread

1 cup fresh berries, such as blueberries and raspberries

4 teaspoons dairy-free butter, such as Earth Balance Buttery Spread, for serving

2 tablespoons toasted sliced almonds

2 tablespoons powdered sugar

Per Serving Calories: 408; Total Carbohydrates: 42g; Sugar: 13g; Total Fat: 22g; Saturated Fat: 8g; Sodium: 397mg; Protein: 11g; Fiber: 4g

1. Preheat the oven to 350°F. Coat the interior of a casserole dish with oil.

2. In a wide, shallow bowl, whisk together the eggs, nut milk, and cinnamon.

3. Dredge the bread slices in the egg mixture. Lay them in the casserole dish, overlapping slightly. Spread the berries over the toast.

4. Bake for 25 to 30 minutes until golden brown.

5. Shower the French toast with powdered sugar and top with sliced almonds. Serve with the dairy-free butter.

SUBSTITUTION TIP: To make this nut-free, substitute another plant-based milk for the nut milk and omit the sliced almonds.

VARIATION TIP: For extra richness, use Cashew Cream (page 22) in the batter instead of the nut milk.

WAFFLES WITH STRAWBERRIES AND WHIPPED CREAM

Nut-Free, Vegetarian

SERVES 4

PREP TIME: 10 minutes COOK TIME: 15 minutes

Doesn't this sound luscious? It is! I've found that the protein and fat in soy milk mimics dairy milk more closely and works better in this recipe than other plant-based milks. It is also usually made with butter, which provides the crisp texture that makes waffles so delectable, but I've opted for coconut or canola oil here. Melted dairy-free butter also works.

For the waffles

1¼ cups all-purpose flour

1 tablespoon sugar

1½ teaspoons baking powder

½ teaspoon sea salt

1 cup Soy Milk (page 23)

⅓ cup coconut oil or canola oil, plus 1 teaspoon

1 egg, whisked

For the whipped cream

½ cup store-bought coconut cream, chilled

1 teaspoon sugar

¼ teaspoon vanilla extract

For the topping

1 pint strawberries, hulled and thinly sliced

Per Serving Calories: 586; Total Carbohydrates: 49g; Sugar: 9g; Total Fat: 41g; Saturated Fat: 32g; Sodium: 253mg; Protein: 8g; Fiber: 3g

Preheat the oven to 200°F.

To make the waffles

1. In a mixing bowl, combine the flour, sugar, baking powder, and salt. Whisk in the soy milk, ⅓ cup of oil, and the egg until just combined.

2. Preheat the waffle iron. Brush with some of the remaining 1 teaspoon of oil.

3. Pour about ½ cup of batter into the waffle maker. Depending on its size, more or less batter may be needed. Cook until browned, place on an oven-safe dish, and transfer to the oven to keep warm.

4. Repeat with the remaining batter, adding more oil to the waffle maker as needed.

continued ☞

To make the whipped cream

While the waffles are cooking, in a small bowl, whip the coconut cream with the sugar and vanilla until thick and creamy.

To serve

To serve, place a waffle on a serving plate, and top with a generous heap of strawberries and a spoonful of whipped cream.

INGREDIENT TIP: This whipped cream mixture can be used in so many different desserts, so keep it in mind for topping Apple Pie (page 179) and Peach Cobbler (page 178). You can purchase coconut cream in a can, or refrigerate a can of regular coconut milk and scoop off the top layer of cream to use in this recipe.

CREAMY VEGETABLE STRATA

Make Gluten-Free, Make Nut-Free, Vegetarian

SERVES 6

PREP TIME: 10 minutes COOK TIME: 25 minutes

This hearty breakfast casserole is loaded with flavor and complex carbohydrates. Use whatever vegetables you have on hand; just make sure they're precooked or safe to eat after minimal cooking. When the strata bakes, it warms and softens the vegetables, but there is insufficient time to cook some foods (for example, raw potatoes).

1 tablespoon canola oil

8 eggs

1 cup Plain Nut Milk (page 20) or Soy Milk (page 23)

½ teaspoon sea salt

¼ teaspoon freshly ground black pepper

2 slices wheat bread or gluten-free bread, crusts removed, cut into cubes, toasted

8 ounces dairy-free cream cheese, cut into cubes (optional)

1 cup frozen broccoli, thawed

½ cup frozen corn, thawed

1 red bell pepper, finely diced

2 tablespoons minced fresh basil or parsley

Per Serving Calories: 159; Total Carbohydrates: 10g; Sugar: 2g; Total Fat: 9g; Saturated Fat: 2g; Sodium: 320mg; Protein: 10g; Fiber: 2g

1. Preheat the oven to 400°F. Coat the interior of a 2-quart casserole dish with the oil.

2. In a large measuring cup, whisk together the eggs, nut milk, salt, and pepper.

3. Spread the toasted bread cubes, dairy-free cream cheese (if using), broccoli, corn, bell pepper, and basil in the casserole dish. Pour the egg mixture over the top, and gently stir to evenly distribute the ingredients.

4. Bake, uncovered, for 20 to 25 minutes, or until the eggs are set and the top is lightly browned. Allow to rest for 5 minutes before serving.

INGREDIENT TIP: If you're using store-bought milk, make sure it is plain and unsweetened. Sweet, vanilla-scented milk doesn't work in this savory casserole.

SKILLET DUTCH BABIES

Make Gluten-Free, Nut-Free, Vegetarian

SERVES 6

PREP TIME: 5 minutes   COOK TIME: 20 minutes

These one-pan oven pancakes offer a convenient way to serve pancakes without all the pouring and flipping. To boot, they have much more protein than traditional pancakes, so they'll stay with you longer. If you prepare the batter the night before, this breakfast comes together in a snap in the morning.

1 dozen eggs

1 cup Coconut Milk (page 24)

2 tablespoons brown sugar

¾ cup all-purpose flour or gluten-free flour blend

¼ teaspoon sea salt

1 tablespoon coconut oil or canola oil

2 tablespoons dairy-free butter, such as Earth Balance Buttery Spread, for serving

2 tablespoons maple syrup, for serving

Per Serving Calories: 271; Total Carbohydrates: 20g; Sugar: 8g; Total Fat: 15g; Saturated Fat: 6g; Sodium: 270mg; Protein: 13g; Fiber: 1g

1. Preheat the oven to 400°F.

2. In a blender, combine the eggs, coconut milk, sugar, flour, and salt. Purée until smooth, scraping down the sides of the blender as needed.

3. In a large skillet over high heat, melt the oil. Using a spatula, evenly coat the interior of the skillet with the oil.

4. Pour the egg mixture into the skillet and transfer to the oven. Bake for 20 minutes or until the Dutch babies are golden brown and puffy. Serve with the dairy-free butter and maple syrup.

COOKING TIP: If you're feeling fancy, top the Dutch babies with sliced fruit such as apples, pears, peaches, or fresh berries before baking. It will not rise quite as high, but the added flavor is a nice tradeoff.

FLUFFY BISCUITS AND SAUSAGE GRAVY

Egg-Free, Make Gluten-Free, Nut-Free

SERVES 4

PREP TIME: 15 minutes   COOK TIME: 15 minutes

Forgive me. This isn't exactly health food, but sometimes you just crave fluffy biscuits and creamy, rich sausage gravy! The lemon juice might sound strange in the biscuits, but go with me. It reacts with the baking soda to leaven the biscuits.

For the biscuits

1 cup all-purpose flour or gluten-free flour blend, plus more for dusting

2 teaspoons aluminum-free baking powder

¼ teaspoon baking soda

½ teaspoon sea salt

¼ cup very cold dairy-free butter, such as Earth Balance Buttery Spread, cut into small cubes

1 teaspoon freshly squeezed lemon juice

⅓ cup Plain Nut Milk (page 20)

For the gravy

8 ounces garlic pork sausage, casings removed, crumbled

2 tablespoons all-purpose flour or gluten-free flour blend

1½ cups plain, unsweetened Soy Milk (page 23)

Sea salt

Freshly ground black pepper

Per Serving Calories: 449; Total Carbohydrates: 30g; Sugar: 1g; Total Fat: 30g; Saturated Fat: 13g; Sodium: 964mg; Protein: 15g; Fiber: 3g

To make the biscuits

1. Preheat the oven to 425°F. Line a sheet pan with parchment paper.

2. In a food processor, combine the flour, baking powder, baking soda, and salt. Add the dairy-free butter, and pulse until small chunks remain.

3. Mix the lemon juice into the nut milk, and pour the milk into the food processor. Pulse once or twice, scraping down the sides as needed, until the dough just comes together.

4. On a clean countertop, spread a layer of flour, and transfer the dough to the floured surface. Gently pat the dough into a large circle or rectangle about ¾- to 1-inch thick.

5. Use a round drinking glass or cookie cutter to cut the dough into biscuits, and transfer them to the sheet pan. Gently reshape the dough and repeat until all the dough is used. You should have about 4 biscuits.

6. Bake for 12 to 14 minutes, until the biscuits are gently browned and puffy.

continued ☞

To make the gravy

1. While the biscuits bake, heat a large skillet over medium heat. Cook the sausage until lightly browned and just cooked through, about 5 minutes.

2. Sprinkle the flour over the skillet, and with a wooden spoon, scrape up the browned bits. Cook for about 1 minute or until the flour has absorbed the fat.

3. Pour in the soy milk and season with salt and pepper. Cook, stirring frequently, until thickened and bubbling. Remove from the heat.

To serve, slice the biscuits in half, and top with a generous spoonful of gravy.

INGREDIENT TIP: For even better results, freeze the butter in small cubes. This keeps it from fully mixing into the biscuit dough, which produces a flakier result.

TEX-MEX BREAKFAST BURRITOS

Make Gluten-Free, Nut-Free, Vegetarian

SERVES 4

PREP TIME: 10 minutes COOK TIME: 10 minutes

As its name suggests, Tex-Mex is a fusion of Texan and Mexican cuisine, characterized by heavy use of shredded cheese, beans, ground meat, sautéed onions and peppers, and spices. This version skips the cheese and meat for a healthy, flavorful, veggie-packed breakfast burrito.

1 tablespoon canola oil

1 green bell pepper, cored and thinly sliced

1 small yellow onion, halved and thinly sliced

1 teaspoon ground cumin

Sea salt

Freshly ground black pepper

6 eggs, whisked

1 cup chili beans, drained, warmed

2 tablespoons minced fresh cilantro

4 flour tortillas

¼ cup Dairy-Free Sour Cream (page 192) or store-bought

½ cup guacamole

Hot sauce, such as Cholula, for serving

Per Serving Calories: 380; Total Carbohydrates: 34g; Sugar: 6g; Total Fat: 22g; Saturated Fat: 4g; Sodium: 657mg; Protein: 15g; Fiber: 8g

1. In a large skillet over medium-high heat, heat the oil. Sauté the pepper and onion until lightly browned and soft, about 5 minutes. Stir in the cumin. Season generously with salt and pepper. Transfer to a separate dish.

2. In the same skillet, cook the eggs until just set, 2 to 3 minutes.

3. To assemble the burritos, divide the chili beans, sautéed pepper and onion, eggs, and cilantro between the flour tortillas. Top each with 1 tablespoon of sour cream and 2 tablespoons of guacamole. Season with hot sauce as desired. Fold into a burrito and enjoy immediately.

SUBSTITUTION TIP: To make this gluten-free, purchase gluten-free flour tortillas. Corn tortillas are okay, too, but they are smaller and should be warmed first to prevent breakage.

FARMERS' MARKET HASH

Gluten-Free, Nut-Free, Vegetarian

SERVES 4

PREP TIME: 10 minutes COOK TIME: 45 minutes

I had the opportunity to work with a team to film the making of this breakfast hash, and when we wrapped the shoot, the production team gathered around the pan and absolutely devoured this simple, healthy breakfast. If you don't have Sriracha, use another hot sauce such as Cholula or Tapatio.

2 russet potatoes

2 small sweet potatoes, scrubbed and diced

1 red bell pepper, cored and sliced

1 yellow onion, halved and sliced

Leaves of 1 rosemary sprig, minced

4 tablespoons canola oil, divided

Sea salt

Freshly ground black pepper

1 large tomato, cut into large chunks

4 eggs

Large handful fresh basil leaves

Sriracha, for serving

Per Serving Calories: 432; Total Carbohydrates: 57g; Sugar: 7g; Total Fat: 19g; Saturated Fat: 3g; Sodium: 142mg; Protein: 11g; Fiber: 9g

1. Preheat the oven to 375°F. Line a rimmed sheet pan with parchment paper.

2. Spread the russet potatoes, sweet potatoes, bell pepper, onion, and rosemary on the sheet pan, and drizzle with 3 tablespoons of oil. Using your hands, toss gently to coat. Sprinkle with salt and pepper.

3. Roast uncovered for 30 minutes or until the vegetables are tender and begin to brown on the bottom.

4. Add the tomato to the pan, and roast for another 5 to 10 minutes, until the tomato has shrunken somewhat.

5. Meanwhile, heat a large skillet over medium-high heat. Once hot, add the remaining 1 tablespoon of oil. Allow it to get hot, about 15 seconds.

6. Crack the eggs into the skillet, being careful not to break the yolks. Season with salt and pepper. Cook until the whites are set and browned around the edges, 5 to 7 minutes.

7. Meanwhile, roll the basil leaves into a tight cylinder, and slice with a sharp knife to make a chiffonade. Scatter the basil over the cooked vegetables.

8. To serve, divide the roasted vegetables between serving dishes, and top each with a fried egg. Serve with Sriracha.

SUBSTITUTION TIP: You can use whatever vegetables and herbs you have on hand. Try whatever's in season, such as zucchini, butternut squash, or broccoli.

BLUEBERRY BREAKFAST CAKE

Make Gluten-Free, Nut-Free, Vegetarian

SERVES 6

PREP TIME: 10 minutes   COOK TIME: 40 minutes

This fruit-studded coffee cake is perfect for lazy midmorning brunches or afternoon tea. If blueberries aren't available, you can use diced fresh peaches or raspberries.

Juice of 1 lemon

½ cup Vanilla Nut Milk (page 21)

¾ cup dairy-free butter, such as Earth Balance Buttery Spread, at room temperature, divided

½ cup sugar, plus 2 tablespoons

2 eggs, whisked

1 teaspoon vanilla extract

Zest of 1 lemon

2 cups all-purpose flour or gluten-free flour blend, plus 2 tablespoons

2 teaspoons baking powder

1 teaspoon sea salt

2 cups fresh blueberries

¼ cup old-fashioned rolled oats

Per Serving Calories: 494; Total Carbohydrates: 62g; Sugar: 26g; Total Fat: 25g; Saturated Fat: 7g; Sodium: 572mg; Protein: 7g; Fiber: 3g

1. Preheat the oven to 350°F. Line an 8-by-8-inch baking dish with parchment paper.

2. In a small bowl, combine the lemon juice and nut milk, and set aside to make a mock buttermilk.

3. In a large bowl, beat ½ cup of dairy-free butter with ½ cup of sugar until thick and fluffy. Add the eggs, vanilla, and lemon zest, and beat until just integrated, about 30 seconds.

4. Sift in the flour, baking powder, and salt. Add the lemon–nut milk mixture, and stir until just integrated. Small lumps will remain. Fold in the blueberries.

5. Pour the mixture into the baking dish.

6. In a small bowl, combine the remaining ¼ cup of dairy-free butter, 2 tablespoons of sugar, 2 tablespoons of flour, and the oats. Sprinkle this streusel over the cake.

7. Bake for 40 minutes or until a cake tester inserted in the center comes out clean.

VARIATION TIP: Turn this dish into a classic coffee cake by omitting the blueberries and lemon zest. Add 1 teaspoon ground cinnamon to the cake batter and ½ teaspoon ground cinnamon to the streusel topping.

COCONUT-MANGO PORRIDGE

Egg-Free, Gluten-Free, Vegan

SERVES 4

PREP TIME: 5 minutes, plus 30 minutes to soak

Looking for something a little different? This breakfast pudding has all the taste of the tropics. It also makes a delicious snack or dessert.

½ cup raw cashews, soaked in hot water for at least 30 minutes

½ cup unsweetened grated coconut

1 cup light coconut milk, divided

¼ cup water

2 tablespoons maple syrup, plus more as desired

2 tablespoons freshly squeezed lime juice

Pinch sea salt

2 tablespoons coconut oil

2 cups diced mango

Per Serving Calories: 428; Total Carbohydrates: 32g; Sugar: 21g; Total Fat: 34g; Saturated Fat: 29g; Sodium: 75mg; Protein: 4g; Fiber: 7g

1. Rinse and drain the cashews. Put them in a blender with the coconut and ½ cup of coconut milk. Blend until smooth, adding only as much water as needed to keep the blender moving.

2. When the cashews are completely smooth, add the remaining ½ cup of coconut milk, the maple syrup, lime juice, and salt.

3. With the motor still running, pour in the oil and blend until thoroughly integrated.

4. Divide the mixture between four small ramekins or glass jars.

5. Clean the blender thoroughly, then add the mango and purée until smooth. Pour over the coconut puddings.

SUBSTITUTION TIP: For a sweet treat, swap the puréed mango for Lemon Curd (page 181).

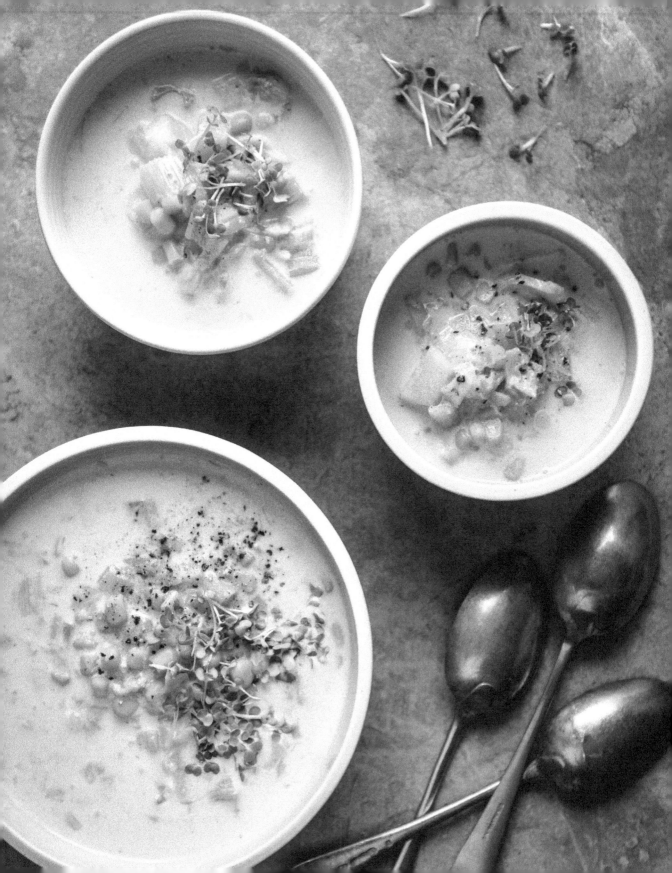

Chapter Five

SALADS AND SOUPS

TOMATO, MINT, AND SHALLOT SALAD

Egg-Free, Gluten-Free, Make Allergen-Free, Nut-Free, Vegan

SERVES 4

PREP TIME: 5 minutes, plus 10 minutes to rest

One summer I worked in the school garden at my kids' school, and our tomato plants were out of control. At one point, there were about 60 ripe beefsteak tomatoes growing. I took several of them home and had to find creative but easy ways of using them up. This salad was one of my favorites that season.

4 large heirloom tomatoes, cored and cut into 1-inch chunks

Leaves of 2 mint sprigs, thinly sliced

1 large shallot, thinly sliced lengthwise

1 tablespoon extra-virgin olive oil

2 teaspoons red wine vinegar

Sea salt

Freshly ground black pepper

Per Serving Calories: 70; Total Carbohydrates: 9g; Sugar: 5g; Total Fat: 4g; Saturated Fat: 1g; Sodium: 71mg; Protein: 2g; Fiber: 3g

1. In a small, nonreactive bowl, combine the tomatoes, mint, shallot, oil, and vinegar. Season generously with salt and pepper.

2. Allow to rest at room temperature for 5 to 10 minutes to allow the flavors to come together.

VARIATION TIP: This salad also works well with fresh basil instead of mint and balsamic vinegar instead of red wine vinegar, capturing the flavors of caprese.

SPICY CITRUS KALE SALAD

Egg-Free, Gluten-Free, Make Allergen-Free, Nut-Free, Vegan

SERVES 4

PREP TIME: 10 minutes

I'm so head over heels in love with this salad. The bracing acidity of the citrus juice and zest, savory garlic, and spicy sambal oelek in the dressing are a surprising and delightful complement to sturdy, mildly sweet kale.

Zest of 1 orange

Zest and juice of 1 lime

1 garlic clove, minced

1 tablespoon canola oil

1 tablespoon extra-virgin olive oil

1 teaspoon sambal oelek (see Ingredient tip)

1 teaspoon maple syrup or honey

¼ teaspoon sea salt

1 bunch fresh kale, stemmed, leaves roughly chopped

2 scallions, thinly sliced on a bias

Per Serving Calories: 118; Total Carbohydrates: 13g; Sugar: 2g; Total Fat: 7g; Saturated Fat: 1g; Sodium: 170mg; Protein: 3g; Fiber: 1g

1. In a small jar, combine the orange zest, lime zest and juice, garlic, canola oil, olive oil, sambal oelek, maple syrup, and salt. Seal the jar tightly, and shake to combine.

2. In a large serving bowl, combine the kale and scallions. Drizzle the dressing over the greens, and use your hands to massage the kale until gently wilted, about 30 seconds.

INGREDIENT TIP: Sambal oelek, made from red chiles, vinegar, and salt, is inexpensive and available in the Asian section of the grocery store or online.

VARIATION TIP: If you can find them, add several thinly sliced kumquats to this salad. They're sweet and tart and can also be eaten whole.

CAESAR SALAD

Make Allergen-Free, Make Egg-Free, Make Gluten-Free, Make Vegan, Nut-Free

SERVES 4

PREP TIME: 5 minutes

A dairy-free Caesar salad is easier to make than you might think. Preparing the dressing from scratch allows you to omit the Parmesan and enjoy a safe and healthy Caesar. Top it with Plant-Based Parmesan and some croutons for a little crunch.

3 garlic cloves, minced

1 teaspoon anchovy paste (optional)

1 teaspoon Worcestershire sauce

½ teaspoon Dijon mustard

1 tablespoon freshly squeezed lemon juice

⅓ cup mayonnaise

2 tablespoons extra-virgin olive oil

Sea salt

Freshly ground black pepper

2 heads romaine lettuce, roughly chopped

1 cup croutons (optional)

¼ cup Plant-Based Parmesan (page 27, optional)

Per Serving Calories: 188; Total Carbohydrates: 13g; Sugar: 3g; Total Fat: 14g; Saturated Fat: 2g; Sodium: 300mg; Protein: 4g; Fiber: 1g

1. In a large mixing bowl, whisk the garlic, anchovy paste (if using), Worcestershire sauce, mustard, lemon juice, and mayonnaise. Slowly drizzle in the oil, whisking constantly. Season with salt and pepper.

2. Add the romaine lettuce to the bowl, and use tongs to toss the salad until well coated. Before serving, top with the croutons (if using) and plant-based Parmesan (if using).

SUBSTITUTION TIP: To make a vegan, egg-free, and allergen-free version of this salad dressing, omit the anchovy paste and use a blend of vegan mayonnaise and Worcestershire sauce.

ASIAN COLD NOODLE SALAD

Egg-Free, Make Gluten-Free, Vegan

SERVES 4

PREP TIME: 10 minutes COOK TIME: 10 minutes

This is one of my family's favorite summer-time dinners. The sweet, spicy, savory Asian dressing coats the chilled noodles and crunchy vegetables and pleases the palate. Add chicken, tofu, or another protein to make this a complete meal.

12 ounces spaghetti noodles

¼ cup soy sauce

1 teaspoon minced ginger

1 teaspoon minced garlic

1 teaspoon sambal oelek (see Ingredient tip on page 53) or pinch red pepper flakes

Juice of 2 limes

1 teaspoon maple syrup or honey

1 tablespoon natural peanut butter

1 small cucumber, peeled, seeded, diced

1 cup sugar snap peas, stringed and halved

½ cup roughly chopped fresh mint

½ cup roughly chopped fresh cilantro

½ cup toasted peanuts, roughly chopped

Per Serving Calories: 488; Total Carbohydrates: 78g; Sugar: 8g; Total Fat: 13g; Saturated Fat: 2g; Sodium: 910mg; Protein: 18g; Fiber: 7g

1. Cook the spaghetti noodles according to the package directions, being careful not to overcook. Rinse under cool running water and drain thoroughly.

2. In a small jar, combine the soy sauce, ginger, garlic, sambal oelek, lime juice, maple syrup, and peanut butter. Seal the jar tightly, and shake vigorously to combine.

3. In a serving bowl, combine the chilled noodles, cucumber, snap peas, mint, and cilantro. Drizzle with the soy-ginger dressing, and toss gently to coat.

4. Before serving, top with the toasted peanuts.

   SUBSTITUTION TIP: To make this dish gluten-free, use gluten-free soy sauce and noodles.

   SUBSTITUTION TIP: For a different spin, use cashew or almond butter and top the dish with roughly chopped roasted cashews.

ROASTED SWEET POTATO SALAD

Egg-Free, Gluten-Free, Vegetarian

SERVES 4

PREP TIME: 10 minutes COOK TIME: 25 minutes

This recipe is adapted from one of my favorite restaurants in LA, Lemonade, a sunny, fresh, cafeteria-style restaurant serving seasonal California cuisine. I worked at an office around the corner in Venice and loved to walk over for lunch.

1 pound sweet potatoes, scrubbed and cut into 1-inch cubes

4 tablespoons extra-virgin olive oil, divided

Sea salt

2 tablespoons sherry vinegar

1 teaspoon freshly squeezed orange juice

1 teaspoon honey

1 small shallot, minced

Freshly ground black pepper

¼ cup minced fresh parsley

¼ cup shelled, roughly chopped pistachios

Per Serving Calories: 284; Total Carbohydrates: 35g; Sugar: 2g; Total Fat: 16g; Saturated Fat: 2g; Sodium: 92mg; Protein: 3g; Fiber: 5g

1. Preheat the oven to 400°F. Line a rimmed sheet pan with parchment paper.

2. Spread the sweet potatoes out on the pan, and toss with 1½ tablespoons of oil. Season with salt. Roast for 25 minutes or until the sweet potatoes are shrunken and lightly browned.

3. Meanwhile, in a small jar, combine the remaining 2½ tablespoons of oil, the sherry vinegar, orange juice, honey, and shallot. Seal tightly and shake to mix. Season with salt and pepper.

4. Allow the sweet potatoes to cool to room temperature. Transfer them to a serving dish.

5. Toss with the parsley and dressing, top with the pistachios, and serve.

INGREDIENT TIP: Honey helps emulsify salad dressings when you're using less oil, as in this vinaigrette.

SOUTHWESTERN CHICKEN SALAD WITH CHIPOTLE RANCH

Gluten-Free, Nut-Free

SERVES 4

PREP TIME: 15 minutes COOK TIME: 10 minutes

This entrée salad is perfect for dinner or a nice lunch. Each of the components can be prepared ahead of time for easy assembly later. I love the chipotle ranch. It is perfectly creamy, spicy, and addicting.

2 (6-ounce) boneless, skinless chicken breasts

1 teaspoon smoked paprika

1 teaspoon ground cumin

Sea salt

Freshly ground black pepper

1 tablespoon canola oil

1 head romaine lettuce, roughly chopped

¼ cup roughly chopped fresh cilantro

1 cup rinsed, drained black beans

1 large tomato, diced

1 avocado, thinly sliced

1 cup frozen corn, thawed

1 to 2 teaspoons minced chipotle in adobo sauce

½ cup Ranch Dressing (page 188)

Per Serving Calories: 343; Total Carbohydrates: 27g; Sugar: 4g; Total Fat: 16g; Saturated Fat: 3g; Sodium: 381mg; Protein: 27g; Fiber: 10g

1. Between two pieces of parchment or wax paper, pound the chicken breasts to a uniform ½-inch thickness. Season with the paprika, cumin, salt, and pepper.

2. In a large skillet over medium-high heat, heat the oil. When it is hot, sear the chicken for about 4 minutes on each side, or until lightly browned and cooked through. Transfer to a cutting board to rest.

3. To assemble the salad, divide the romaine lettuce, cilantro, black beans, tomato, avocado, and corn between serving bowls.

4. Whisk the chipotle into the ranch dressing, adding more chipotle as desired for greater spice.

5. Slice the chicken breasts into thin strips and lay them on the salads. Drizzle each salad with the chipotle ranch.

    SERVING TIP: For a little crunch, top each salad with a tablespoon of toasted pepitas.

STRAWBERRY-SPINACH SALAD

Egg-Free, Gluten-Free, Vegan

SERVES 4

PREP TIME: 5 minutes

Cool, creamy soft cheese is a wonderful complement to many green salads. Fortunately, nut cheese works really well in place of goat cheese, feta, and other soft cheeses. It serves as the "icing on the cake" for this colorful and health-supportive salad.

8 cups baby spinach

1 pint strawberries, hulled and sliced

½ small red onion, thinly sliced

¼ cup Balsamic Vinaigrette (page 186)

½ cup Basic Nut Cheese (page 28)

Per Serving Calories: 115; Total Carbohydrates: 11g; Sugar: 6g; Total Fat: 7g; Saturated Fat: 1g; Sodium: 184mg; Protein: 3g; Fiber: 4g

1. In a large bowl, combine the spinach, strawberries, and onion. Add the balsamic vinaigrette, tossing gently to coat the leaves in the dressing.

2. Divide the salad between serving plates.

3. Add the nut cheese in bite-size chunks over the salad. Serve immediately.

SUBSTITUTION TIP: If you're short on time but want the creamy nut cheese, opt for a store-bought variety such as Treeline or Miyoko's Creamery.

SERVING TIP: This cheese will keep, covered, for up to 5 days in the refrigerator.

CURRIED LENTIL SOUP WITH CILANTRO SALSA

Allergen-Free, Egg-Free, Gluten-Free, Nut-Free, Vegan

SERVES 4

PREP TIME: 10 minutes   COOK TIME: 25 minutes

This is my all-time favorite lentil soup. It's not at all traditional, but the flavors are so good, I keep coming back. The recipe is adapted from the vegan restaurant Vedge in Philadelphia. The soup served as one of my staples when I was training for a half marathon over the winter. I came in from long runs with bright red cheeks and a deep hunger for its spicy, warming goodness.

1 small red onion, finely diced

1 cup minced fresh cilantro

2 scallions, thinly sliced on a bias

1 teaspoon sea salt plus more for seasoning

Juice of 1 lemon

1 tablespoon canola oil

1 yellow onion, minced

1 teaspoon minced fresh ginger

1 tablespoon yellow curry powder

1 cup green lentils, picked over

8 cups vegetable broth

Freshly ground black pepper

Per Serving Calories: 303; Total Carbohydrates: 36g; Sugar: 5g; Total Fat: 7g; Saturated Fat: 1g; Sodium: 2004mg; Protein: 23g; Fiber: 16g

1. In a large glass jar, combine the red onion, cilantro, scallions, salt, and lemon juice. Seal tightly, and shake to combine. Refrigerate for at least 30 minutes.

2. In a large pot over medium heat, heat the oil. Add the onion and ginger, and cook, stirring occasionally, for 5 minutes. Add the curry powder, and cook for another minute.

3. Add the lentils and vegetable broth, and bring to a simmer. Cover and simmer for 20 minutes.

4. Transfer 2 cups of soup to a blender, vent the lid, and place a kitchen towel over it to protect from spattering (see Cooking tip). Carefully purée until smooth. Return the puréed soup to the pot, and season with salt and pepper.

5. Divide the soup between serving bowls, and top with the onion and cilantro salsa.

COOKING TIP: Use an immersion blender to avoid the risk of your blender exploding all over with hot soup.

CREAMY TORTILLA SOUP

Egg-Free, Gluten-Free, Make Allergen-Free, Make Nut-Free

SERVES 4

PREP TIME: 10 minutes COOK TIME: 15 minutes

If you're a soup enthusiast like I am, you probably know how much fun it is to turn an everyday dinner item such as tacos into a comforting soup. While I'm certainly not the first to do this, I did have to think outside the box a bit to make a satisfyingly rich and creamy dairy-free tortilla soup. I hope you'll love this version as much as I do.

1 tablespoon canola oil

1 red onion, diced

1 green bell pepper, diced

3 garlic cloves, minced

1 teaspoon ground cumin

1 teaspoon ground paprika

1 pound lean ground beef

Sea salt

Freshly ground black pepper

4 cups chicken broth

1 cup frozen corn, thawed

½ cup Cashew Cream (page 22)

2 tablespoons freshly squeezed lime juice, plus lime wedges, for serving

4 cups blue corn tortilla chips, for serving

Per Serving Calories: 431; Total Carbohydrates: 27g; Sugar: 4g; Total Fat: 20g; Saturated Fat: 6g; Sodium: 1008mg; Protein: 32g; Fiber: 4g

1. In a large pot over medium-high heat, heat the oil. Sauté the onion and bell pepper for 3 to 4 minutes, until they begin to soften.

2. Add the garlic, cumin, and paprika. Cook for 1 minute.

3. Push the vegetables to the side and crumble the ground beef into the center of the pot. Season with salt and pepper. Cook until lightly browned and just cooked through.

4. Add the chicken broth to the pot, and simmer for 5 minutes. Stir in the corn, cashew cream, and lime juice, and cook for 2 more minutes.

5. Serve with the lime wedges and tortilla chips.

SUBSTITUTION TIP: For an allergen-free, nut-free version, skip the cashew cream and stir in ½ cup Dairy-Free Sour Cream (page 192) or the store-bought version.

CORN CHOWDER

Egg-Free, Gluten-Free, Nut-Free, Vegan

SERVES 4

PREP TIME: 10 minutes COOK TIME: 35 minutes

Freshly shucked corn is a must in this dairy-free corn chowder that's perfect for late summer lunches. The starch of the potato adds nice body and a creamy texture. The dairy-free sour cream infuses a bit of tang and even more creaminess for an absolutely decadent soup.

1 tablespoon canola oil

1 medium leek, washed thoroughly, diced

1 yellow onion, diced

Sea salt

1 russet potato, peeled and finely diced

4 thyme sprigs

4 cups vegetable broth

4 ears corn on the cob, kernels removed (reserve ½ cup kernels, for serving)

1 tablespoon white wine vinegar

½ cup Dairy-Free Sour Cream (page 192) or store-bought

Freshly ground black pepper

2 scallions, green parts only, thinly sliced

1 tablespoon extra-virgin olive oil, for drizzling

Handful microgreens or sprouts (optional)

Per Serving Calories: 352; Total Carbohydrates: 46g; Sugar: 10g; Total Fat: 16g; Saturated Fat: 7g; Sodium: 884mg; Protein: 12g; Fiber: 6g

1. In a medium pot, heat the canola oil over medium heat. Reduce the heat to low, and add the leek and onion with a generous pinch salt to help the vegetables release their liquids. Cook for about 15 minutes, until soft and pulpy.

2. Add the potato, thyme, vegetable broth, corncobs, and corn kernels. Cook for a further 15 to 20 minutes.

3. Remove and discard the corncobs and thyme.

4. Stir in the vinegar, then add the dairy-free sour cream.

5. Using an immersion blender, purée the soup until smooth. Season with salt and pepper.

6. Pour the soup into wide soup bowls. Garnish with the scallions, reserved corn kernels, olive oil, microgreens (if using), and a grind of pepper.

SUBSTITUTION TIP: To make this soy-free, you can substitute the non-dairy sour cream with ½ cup of non-dairy plain coffee creamer, such as So Delicious Dairy Free Original Coconutmilk Creamer.

WHITE GAZPACHO

Egg-Free, Gluten-Free, Vegan

SERVES 4

PREP TIME: 10 minutes, plus 30 minutes to chill

You might be thinking, how could white gazpacho ever compete with the tangy, refreshing tomato soup you know and love? Rename this one if you like, but definitely give it a try. The chilled almond milk broth is creatively studded with green grapes, chives, and cucumbers.

4 cups peeled and diced cucumber, divided

3 cups green grapes, divided

2 garlic cloves, minced

1 cup Plain Nut Milk (page 20) made with almonds

2 tablespoons extra-virgin olive oil

1 tablespoon sherry vinegar

Sea salt

Freshly ground black pepper

¼ cup slivered almonds, toasted, for serving

4 fresh chives, chopped, for serving

Per Serving Calories: 170; Total Carbohydrates: 18g; Sugar: 13g; Total Fat: 11g; Saturated Fat: 1g; Sodium: 108mg; Protein: 3g; Fiber: 2g

1. In a blender, combine 3½ cups of cucumber, 2½ cups of grapes, the garlic, nut milk, oil, and vinegar. Purée until smooth. Season with salt and pepper.

2. For a smoother soup, pass through a China cap or fine mesh strainer.

3. Pour the soup into a container, cover, and chill the soup thoroughly in the refrigerator about 30 minutes. Before serving, shake the container vigorously if the soup has separated.

4. To serve, pour the chilled soup into individual serving bowls, and top with the remaining ½ cup of cucumber, ½ cup of grapes, the slivered almonds, and chives.

SUBSTITUTION TIP: If you don't have sherry vinegar, white wine vinegar or champagne vinegar will also work.

TOM YUM COCONUT SOUP

Egg-Free, Gluten-Free, Nut-Free

SERVES 4

PREP TIME: 10 minutes COOK TIME: 15 minutes

My first taste of Tom Yum soup was at an authentic Thai restaurant and laundromat in north Portland. The spicy, tangy, and floral broth captivated me, and I was eager to recreate it at home. Asian markets abound in Portland, so finding the lemongrass, kaffir, and galangal there was easy, but I know that isn't true of every town, so in this version, I call for Tom Yum paste. If you want to make your own, see the Ingredient tip. This soup is delicious with steamed white rice and a simple side salad.

1 tablespoon canola oil

1 pound boneless, skinless chicken breast, cut into 2-inch pieces

1 onion, halved and thinly sliced

4 cups chicken broth

2 tablespoons Tom Yum paste

2 plum tomatoes, cored and diced

1 cup button mushrooms, quartered

1 teaspoon sugar

2 tablespoons fish sauce

3 tablespoons freshly squeezed lime juice

1 cup full-fat coconut milk

Sea salt

Freshly ground black pepper

1 cup roughly chopped fresh cilantro

2 scallions, thinly sliced on a bias

Per Serving Calories: 398; Total Carbohydrates: 13g; Sugar: 7g; Total Fat: 24g; Saturated Fat: 14g; Sodium: 1980mg; Protein: 32g; Fiber: 3g

1. In a large pot over medium-high heat, heat the oil. Add the chicken and onion, and sauté for 10 minutes.

2. Add the chicken broth, Tom Yum paste, tomatoes, and mushrooms, and cook for 5 minutes, until the chicken is cooked through and the vegetables are soft.

3. Stir in the sugar, fish sauce, lime juice, and coconut milk, and simmer for 1 minute. Season with salt and pepper.

4. Just before serving, stir in the cilantro and scallions.

INGREDIENT TIP: You can find Tom Yum paste in the Asian section of most grocery stores or order it online. To make your own, use a mortar and pestle to mash 1 tablespoon of minced lemongrass, 1 teaspoon of minced galangal root, 4 shredded kaffir lime leaves, and 2 Thai chiles.

CREAMY TOMATO SOUP

Egg-Free, Gluten-Free, Make Vegan

SERVES 4

PREP TIME: 5 minutes COOK TIME: 15 minutes

One of my earliest food memories is of tomato soup and grilled cheese sandwiches in the second grade. Fast-forward a few decades, my children are in elementary school, and the combo is still a classic favorite. This creamy tomato soup is thickened with cashew cream, and it pairs like a charm with a grilled cheese sandwich made with a dairy-free Cheddar cheese such as Follow Your Heart.

2 tablespoons extra-virgin olive oil

3 garlic cloves, minced

2 shallots, thinly sliced

Pinch red pepper flakes

1 (28-ounce) can plum tomatoes, crushed, with juices

½ cup roughly chopped fresh basil, plus more for serving

2 cups chicken broth

½ cup Cashew Cream (page 22), plus 2 tablespoons

Sea salt

Freshly ground black pepper

Per Serving Calories: 192; Total Carbohydrates: 12g; Sugar: 7g; Total Fat: 15g; Saturated Fat: 8g; Sodium: 455mg; Protein: 5g; Fiber: 3g

1. In a large pot over medium-low heat, heat the oil. Add the garlic, shallots, red pepper flakes, tomatoes and their juices, and basil, and cook for 10 minutes, until soft and pulpy.

2. Pour in the broth, and bring to a gentle simmer for 5 minutes.

3. Remove the soup from the heat, and allow to cool for 5 minutes. Purée with an immersion blender. For a very smooth soup, pass it through a China cap or fine mesh strainer.

4. Whisk in ½ cup of cashew cream. Season with salt and pepper.

5. To serve, divide the soup between serving bowls, and swirl in the remaining 2 table-spoons of cashew cream. Garnish each bowl with the additional basil.

SUBSTITUTION TIP: To make this soup vegan, use vegetable broth in place of the chicken broth.

CREAM OF MUSHROOM SOUP

Egg-Free, Gluten-Free, Make Allergen-Free, Make Vegan, Nut-Free

SERVES 4

PREP TIME: 10 minutes COOK TIME: 17 minutes

If you didn't think cream of mushroom soup was possible without cream, you're in for a surprise. Typically, I use cashew cream or dairy-free sour cream to thicken the soup and give it that creamy consistency, but this time I'm opting for white beans and dairy-free butter.

1 tablespoon canola oil

4 tablespoons dairy-free butter, such as Earth Balance Buttery Spread, divided

2 cups sliced mushrooms

1 small yellow onion, diced

2 garlic cloves, minced

1 teaspoon minced fresh thyme leaves

2 tablespoons sherry

1½ quarts chicken broth or vegetable broth

1 cup canned white beans, such as cannellini, rinsed and drained

Sea salt

Freshly ground black pepper

Per Serving Calories: 277; Total Carbohydrates: 17g; Sugar: 3g; Total Fat: 17g; Saturated Fat: 4g; Sodium: 1424mg; Protein: 12g; Fiber: 6g

1. In a wide, deep skillet over medium-high heat, heat the oil and 1 tablespoon of dairy-free butter. Add a handful of mushrooms to the skillet, and cook for 1 to 2 minutes on each side. Push the cooked mushrooms to the side, and repeat until all the mushrooms are used.

2. Add the onion, garlic, and thyme to the skillet, and cook, stirring occasionally, for another 5 minutes.

3. Pour the sherry into the skillet, and cook off the alcohol, about 1 minute. Add the broth, and bring to a simmer for 1 minute.

4. Transfer 2 cups of soup to a blender, and add the white beans. Purée until very smooth. Return the soup to the skillet, and bring to a simmer for 1 minute.

5. Whisk in the remaining 3 tablespoons of dairy-free butter, and season with salt and pepper.

INGREDIENT TIP: For an even richer mushroom flavor, soak 1 ounce of dried wild mushrooms in 1 cup of boiling water for 10 minutes. Strain the mushrooms, reserving the liquid and discarding any sediment. Roughly chop the mushrooms and add them to the soup just before adding the sherry. Add the mushroom broth to the soup with the other broth in place of 1 cup of broth.

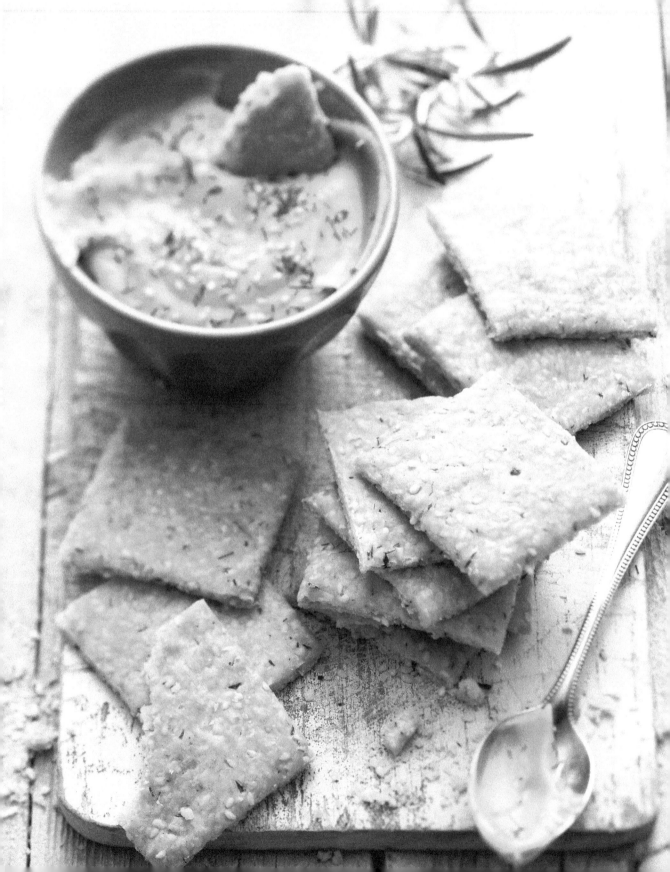

Chapter Six

SNACKS AND SIDES

FRUIT AND NUT BARS

Egg-Free, Gluten-Free, Vegan

YIELD: 8 bars

PREP TIME: 10 minutes

This basic recipe can be taken in so many different directions and is an essential part of my dairy-free snack repertoire. I love adding dairy-free dark chocolate chips and a splash of vanilla extract for a chocolate chip cookie dough version. Or I'll add cinnamon and orange zest for an autumn-spiced version.

For Healthy Brownie Bars

1¼ cups walnuts

Pinch sea salt

1 cup pitted dates

2 tablespoons cocoa powder

½ teaspoon vanilla extract

For Key Lime Pie Bars

¾ cup raw cashews

½ cup walnuts

Pinch sea salt

1 cup pitted dates

1 teaspoon lime zest

1 teaspoon freshly squeezed lime juice

For Chocolate Chip Cookie Dough Bars

¾ cup walnuts

½ cup raw cashews

Pinch sea salt

1 cup pitted dates

½ cup dairy-free dark chocolate pieces

¼ teaspoon vanilla extract

For Autumn Spice Bars

1¼ cups pecans

Pinch sea salt

1 cup pitted dates

1 teaspoon ground cinnamon

1 teaspoon orange zest

1 teaspoon freshly squeezed orange juice

To make the bars

1. In a food processor, combine the nuts and salt, and pulse until coarsely ground.

2. Add the dates, and process until fully blended.

3. Add the remaining variation add-ins, and blend just until integrated.

4. Spread the mixture out on a clean cutting board. Press and form into a rectangle. Cut into 8 bars. Store in a covered container in the refrigerator.

Healthy Brownie Bars

Per Serving Calories: 99; Total Carbohydrates: 18g; Sugar: 14g; Total Fat: 3g; Saturated Fat: 0g; Sodium: 32mg; Protein: 1g; Fiber: 3g

Key Lime Pie Bars

Per Serving Calories: 134; Total Carbohydrates: 20g; Sugar: 14g; Total Fat: 6g; Saturated Fat: 1g; Sodium: 33mg; Protein: 3g; Fiber: 2g

Chocolate Chip Cookie Dough Bars

Per Serving Calories: 198; Total Carbohydrates: 29g; Sugar: 14g; Total Fat: 9g; Saturated Fat: 3g; Sodium: 32mg; Protein: 3g; Fiber: 2g

Autumn Spice Bars

Per Serving Calories: 95; Total Carbohydrates: 18g; Sugar: 14g; Total Fat: 3g; Saturated Fat: 0g; Sodium: 32mg; Protein: 1g; Fiber: 2g

MARINATED CHICKPEAS

Allergen-Free, Egg-Free, Gluten-Free, Nut-Free, Vegan

SERVES 4

PREP TIME: 10 minutes

Chickpeas are a good source of protein and complex carbohydrates and can be used in so many different recipes. But they can be a little boring straight out of the can. This marinade transforms them into a delicious salad topping, side dish, or quick snack. The ingredient list is a bit long, but be assured, it is mostly pantry and grocery staples, such as oil, vinegar, and carrot, you probably have on hand.

2 tablespoons red wine vinegar

1 tablespoon white wine vinegar

1 tablespoon extra-virgin olive oil

1 garlic clove, minced

1 teaspoon minced fresh thyme leaves or ½ teaspoon dried thyme

1 teaspoon lemon zest

1 carrot, minced

1 celery stalk, minced

1 shallot, minced

Sea salt

Freshly ground black pepper

2 (15-ounce) cans chickpeas, rinsed and drained

Per Serving Calories: 329; Total Carbohydrates: 57g; Sugar: 1g; Total Fat: 6g; Saturated Fat: 1g; Sodium: 791mg; Protein: 12g; Fiber: 11g

1. In a large jar, whisk together the red wine vinegar, white wine vinegar, oil, garlic, thyme, lemon zest, carrot, celery, and shallot. Season generously with salt and pepper.

2. Add the chickpeas to the marinade, seal the jar tightly, and shake gently to combine.

3. Store, covered, in the refrigerator for up to 4 days.

   COOKING TIP: The flavors get even better as the chickpeas sit in the marinade, so if time allows, make it several hours in advance of when you intend to serve it.

CRANBERRY AND CRACKED PEPPER CHEESE BALL

Egg-Free, Gluten-Free, Vegan

SERVES 6

PREP TIME: 5 minutes

Your classic party appetizer is back! And this time it's dairy-free. Sweet, tart cranberries and savory shallots and thyme are the perfect complement to the Basic Nut Cheese.

1 recipe Basic Nut Cheese (page 28) made with cashews or macadamia nuts

2 tablespoons minced shallots

1 tablespoon minced fresh thyme leaves

Sea salt

Freshly ground black pepper

½ cup dried cranberries

Per Serving Calories: 117; Total Carbohydrates: 8g; Sugar: 3g; Total Fat: 8g; Saturated Fat: 1g; Sodium: 66mg; Protein: 3g; Fiber: 1g

1. Place the nut cheese into a nut milk bag or a colander lined with cheesecloth. Squeeze the excess moisture from the nut cheese with your hands, or set the colander over a bowl in the refrigerator and allow it to drain for 30 minutes or until the nut cheese can hold its shape.

2. Place the nut cheese in a clean bowl, and mix in the shallots and thyme. Season with salt and pepper.

3. Form the cheese into a small ball. On a small plate, spread out the dried cranberries, then roll the cheese ball in the cranberries until the ball is covered. Transfer to a serving platter, or cover and refrigerate until ready to serve.

SERVING TIP: Serve with sturdy crackers or vegetable chips.

PISTACHIO AND HERB "GOAT" CHEESE

Egg-Free, Gluten-Free, Vegan

SERVES 6

PREP TIME: 5 minutes

Grassy herbs and sweet, salty pistachios form a delicious crust around the Basic Nut Cheese. A variety of herbs will work in this recipe, so use what you have. I like fresh tarragon, cilantro, and oregano, as well as the trio called for below.

1 recipe Basic Nut Cheese (page 28), made with cashews or macadamia nuts

1 tablespoon minced fresh thyme leaves

1 tablespoon minced fresh basil

1 tablespoon minced fresh parsley

¼ cup finely chopped pistachios

Per Serving Calories: 119; Total Carbohydrates: 6g; Sugar: 0g; Total Fat: 9g; Saturated Fat: 1g; Sodium: 84mg; Protein: 4g; Fiber: 1g

1. Place the nut cheese into a nut milk bag or a colander lined with cheesecloth. Squeeze the excess moisture from the nut cheese with your hands, or set the colander over a bowl in the refrigerator and allow to drain for 30 minutes, or until the nut cheese can hold its shape.

2. On a small plate, mix together the thyme, basil, parsley, and pistachios, and spread it out.

3. Form the cheese into a small log, and roll it in the herb and nut mixture. Transfer to a serving platter, or cover and refrigerate until ready to serve.

SERVING TIP: Serve this cheese with oil-packed sun-dried tomatoes and crostini for a decadent appetizer.

SWEET POTATO HUMMUS

Allergen-Free, Egg-Free, Gluten-Free, Nut-Free, Vegan

YIELD: 2 cups

PREP TIME: 5 minutes COOK TIME: 50 minutes

Let me say first, this sweet potato hummus is nothing like traditional hummus and is only so named because it contains chickpeas. However, it is savory and delicious, and works nicely as a dip for chips or vegetables or in Chipotle Sweet Potato Quesadillas (page 151).

1 medium sweet potato

1 (15-ounce) can chickpeas, rinsed and drained

1 chipotle in adobo, minced

1 teaspoon adobo sauce

2 tablespoons nutritional yeast

2 teaspoons apple cider vinegar

1 teaspoon sugar

½ teaspoon sea salt

Per Serving (¼ cup) Calories: 94; Total Carbohydrates: 18g; Sugar: 1g; Total Fat: 1g; Saturated Fat: 0g; Sodium: 302mg; Protein: 4g; Fiber: 4g

1. Preheat the oven to 400°F. Prick the sweet potato all over with a fork and bake for 50 minutes or until the potato is very tender and syrup oozes from the holes in the skin.

2. Carefully scrape the roasted sweet potato flesh into a blender. Add the chickpeas, chipotle, adobo sauce, yeast, vinegar, sugar, and salt. Purée until smooth, scraping down the sides as needed.

COOKING TIP: Spread a layer of aluminum foil on the oven rack beneath the sweet potato to catch any drips.

POLENTA FRIES

Allergen-Free, Egg-Free, Gluten-Free, Nut-Free, Vegan

SERVES 4

PREP TIME: 10 minutes COOK TIME: 40 to 45 minutes

Creamy polenta is traditionally made with milk and Parmesan and takes at least half an hour to make. But for these oven-fries, the packaged polenta (which is typically dairy-free) is also hassle-free. Even better, the prepared polenta is super easy to slice into fries that are perfect for dipping in savory Pomodoro Sauce.

1 (18-ounce) package prepared, dairy-free polenta

2 tablespoons extra-virgin olive oil

1 tablespoon minced fresh rosemary leaves (optional)

Sea salt

Freshly ground black pepper

1 cup Pomodoro Sauce (page 195) or good-quality store-bought marinara sauce

Per Serving Calories: 204; Total Carbohydrates: 28g; Sugar: 7g; Total Fat: 9g; Saturated Fat: 1g; Sodium: 710mg; Protein: 4g; Fiber: 3g

1. Preheat the oven to 425°F. Line a rimmed sheet pan with parchment paper.

2. Cut the polenta in half cross-wise, then cut into ½- to 1-inch-thick spears. Carefully place the polenta spears on the pan, and drizzle with the oil. Season with the rosemary (if using), salt, and pepper. Turn the spears over to coat in the oil.

3. Bake for 40 to 45 minutes or until golden and crisp on the outside, and serve with the sauce for dipping.

SERVING TIP: Polenta fries also make an excellent side dish for meaty dishes such as Balsamic Pot Roast (page 120) or Bacon-Wrapped Chicken (page 137). If cooking in the same pan, reduce the heat to 400° F.

SPINACH-ARTICHOKE DIP

Egg-Free, Gluten-Free, Vegan

SERVES 6

PREP TIME: 10 minutes, plus at least 30 minutes to soak COOK TIME: 30 minutes

Soaked cashews and creamy silken tofu come together to create a luxurious sauce in this classic chip dip stand-in. It's a party favorite and surprisingly similar to the original. However, with a fraction of the fat and calories of the original, it's an indulgence you can feel good about!

1 tablespoon canola oil

1 yellow onion, diced

4 garlic cloves, minced

1 teaspoon minced fresh thyme or ½ teaspoon dried

Pinch red pepper flakes

2 tablespoons freshly squeezed lemon juice

1 (12-ounce) package silken tofu

½ cup raw cashews, soaked in cold water for 8 hours or hot water for 30 minutes

1 teaspoon garlic powder

½ teaspoon sea salt

¼ to ½ cup water

2 cups roughly chopped spinach

1 (15-ounce) can artichoke hearts, drained, quartered

2 tablespoons Plant-Based Parmesan (page 27, optional)

Per Serving Calories: 157; Total Carbohydrates: 15g; Sugar: 3g; Total Fat: 8g; Saturated Fat: 1g; Sodium: 254mg; Protein: 9g; Fiber: 5g

1. Preheat the oven to 350°F.

2. In a large, oven-safe skillet over medium heat, heat the oil. Add the onion, garlic, thyme, and red pepper flakes, and cook for 5 to 7 minutes.

3. Meanwhile, in a blender, combine the lemon juice, tofu, cashews, garlic powder, and salt. Purée until very smooth, adding only as much water as needed to keep the blender moving. Set aside.

4. Add the spinach to the skillet, and cook until thoroughly wilted and the moisture has evaporated, about 3 minutes.

5. Add the artichoke hearts, and cook until just heated through.

6. Pour the cashew and tofu mixture into the skillet, give everything a good stir, then smooth into an even layer. Top with the plant-based Parmesan (if using), then bake uncovered for 15 to 20 minutes, until the top forms a light crust.

7. Serve with sliced vegetables or chips.

INGREDIENT TIP: Silken tofu is available in the Asian section of the grocery store and is not typically refrigerated. Regular soft tofu can be used in a pinch, but it lacks the creamy texture of silken tofu.

NACHO CHEESE DIP

Egg-Free, Make Gluten-Free, Vegan

SERVES 6

PREP TIME: 5 minutes, plus at least 30 minutes to soak COOK TIME: 30 minutes

This dip is spicy, smoky, and creamy—everything you could want in a nacho cheese dip and nothing you don't. Like the Spinach-Artichoke Dip (page 74), this creamy base is made with cashews and silken tofu. It gets a boost of color and flavor from steamed carrots and cheesy flavor from nutritional yeast.

1 cup diced carrots

1 tablespoon canola oil

1 yellow onion, diced

2 garlic cloves, minced

½ cup raw cashews, soaked in cold water for 8 hours or hot water for 30 minutes

1 (12-ounce) package silken tofu

2 tablespoons nutritional yeast

2 tablespoons freshly squeezed lime juice

1 tablespoon tomato paste

1 to 2 teaspoons minced chipotle in adobo sauce

1 teaspoon smoked paprika

1 teaspoon garlic powder

½ teaspoon ground cumin

½ teaspoon sea salt

¼ to ½ cup water

Per Serving Calories: 141; Total Carbohydrates: 10g; Sugar: 3g; Total Fat: 8g; Saturated Fat: 1g; Sodium: 195mg; Protein: 8g; Fiber: 2g

1. Preheat the oven to 350°F.

2. In a steamer basket set over simmering water, steam the carrots for 5 to 7 minutes, until tender. Transfer them to a blender.

3. While the carrots cook, heat the oil in a large, oven-safe skillet over medium heat. Cook the onion and garlic for 3 to 4 minutes, until beginning to soften.

4. Rinse and drain the cashews, discarding the soaking liquid. Put them in a blender along with the tofu, yeast, lime juice, tomato paste, chipotle, paprika, garlic powder, cumin, and salt. Blend, adding only as much water as needed to keep the blender moving.

5. Pour the cashew and tofu mixture into the skillet, give everything a good stir, then smooth into an even layer. Bake uncovered for 15 to 20 minutes, until the top forms a light crust.

6. Serve with corn tortilla chips.

   INGREDIENT TIP: Chipotle in adobo sauce can be found in the Mexican foods section of the grocery store. Wheat is sometimes added as a thickener, so read the labels carefully if you follow a gluten-free diet.

SPICY JALAPEÑO
BAKED TAQUITOS

Egg-Free, Gluten-Free, Make Allergen-Free, Nut-Free, Vegan

SERVES 4

PREP TIME: 10 minutes COOK TIME: 15 minutes

I cannot express the level of disappointment I felt when I discovered the Trader Joe's black bean taquitos I had just bitten into had cheese in them. They were perfectly crisp on the outside, and savory and spicy on the inside. I just had to create a dairy-free alternative! While you certainly could make the refried beans from scratch with fresh onion, jalapeño, and spices, I wanted a recipe that was almost as easy as the original. The kids love them for snack time, and they're healthier than the original.

12 corn tortillas

1 (15-ounce) can spicy jalapeño or salsa-style refried black beans

2 tablespoons canola oil

1 cup prepared guacamole, for serving

Per Serving Calories: 440; Total Carbohydrates: 49g; Sugar: 3g; Total Fat: 26g; Saturated Fat: 3g; Sodium: 464mg; Protein: 9g; Fiber: 12g

1. Preheat the oven to 425°F.

2. Heat the corn tortillas individually in the microwave for about 10 seconds each to soften.

3. Place 2 generous tablespoons of refried beans in a line down one side of each tortilla, about one-third of the way in from the edge, and roll in a tight cylinder. Place them on a rimmed sheet pan, seam-side down.

4. Brush the tortillas lightly with the oil. Bake for 15 minutes or until the tortillas are crisp and beginning to brown. Allow to cool for a few minutes before serving with the guacamole on the side.

INGREDIENT TIP: If you want to keep these vegan, read the label of the refried beans to ensure they don't contain lard.

SAUTÉED BRUSSELS SPROUTS

Egg-Free, Gluten-Free, Make Allergen-Free, Nut-Free, Vegan

SERVES 4

PREP TIME: 10 minutes COOK TIME: 3 minutes

I first tried this side dish at a tapas restaurant called milk & honey in Santa Barbara. The dish was simple but addictive, and my friend and I polished it off in minutes. I knew I could recreate it at home and was pleasantly surprised at how easy it was.

1 pound Brussels sprouts, trimmed (see Ingredient tip)

2 tablespoons extra-virgin olive oil

2 garlic cloves, minced

2 tablespoons red wine vinegar

1 teaspoon maple syrup or honey

Sea salt

Freshly ground black pepper

Per Serving Calories: 117; Total Carbohydrates: 12g; Sugar: 4g; Total Fat: 8g; Saturated Fat: 1g; Sodium: 88mg; Protein: 4g; Fiber: 4g

1. Carefully shred the Brussels sprouts with the single-blade grater attachment of a food processor.

2. In a large skillet over medium-high heat, heat the oil. Add the garlic, and cook for 30 seconds to mellow out the flavor.

3. Add the Brussels sprouts, and sauté until barely wilted, about 2 minutes. Any longer will result in a bitter flavor.

4. Drizzle with the vinegar and maple syrup, and season with salt and pepper.

   INGREDIENT TIP: To prepare the Brussels sprouts, cut off the tough stem end and remove any discolored outer leaves. Rinse under cold water and drain.

SWEET POTATO CORN CAKES

Make Gluten-Free, Vegetarian

SERVES 4

PREP TIME: 5 minutes COOK TIME: 25 to
30 minutes

These delicious sweet potato cakes fall
somewhere between latkes and corn fritters.
They're spicy and savory and perfectly crisp
on the outside. They pair well with Turkey
Mushroom Stew (page 143).

2 medium sweet
potatoes, grated

1 cup corn kernels

1 teaspoon
smoked paprika

½ teaspoon
ground cumin

¼ cup all-purpose
flour or gluten-free
flour blend

½ teaspoon sea salt

1 egg, whisked

Per Serving Calories: 168; Total Carbohydrates: 35g;
Sugar: 2g; Total Fat: 2g; Saturated Fat: 1g; Sodium: 262mg;
Protein: 5g; Fiber: 5g

1. Preheat the oven to 400°F. Line a sheet
   pan with parchment paper.

2. In a small bowl, mix together the sweet
   potatoes, corn, paprika, cumin, flour, salt,
   and egg.

3. Form the mixture into 8 small patties,
   and place them on the sheet pan.

4. Bake for 25 to 30 minutes or until the
   cakes are crisp on the outside and tender
   on the inside.

VARIATION TIP: You can make these cakes
with any starchy root vegetable, such as
potatoes, parsnips, or turnips.

CREAMY MISO SHIITAKE KALE

Egg-Free, Gluten-Free, Nut-Free, Vegan

SERVES 4

PREP TIME: 5 minutes, plus 10 minutes to soak
COOK TIME: 25 minutes

Creamy stewed greens don't have to become a distant memory in a dairy-free diet. This savory side dish combines the umami, or savory, flavors of miso and mushrooms in a thick coconut cream sauce. The garlic nicely masks any coconut undertones, so no one will ever know it's dairy-free!

½ ounce dried shiitake mushrooms

1 cup hot water, for soaking

1 tablespoon canola oil or extra-virgin olive oil

1 shallot, thinly sliced

3 garlic cloves, minced

Sea salt

2 bunches kale, leaves roughly chopped, stems minced

½ cup full-fat coconut milk

1 tablespoon white miso

½ teaspoon low-sodium soy sauce

¾ teaspoon red wine vinegar

Freshly ground black pepper

Per Serving Calories: 207; Total Carbohydrates: 23g; Sugar: 1g; Total Fat: 11g; Saturated Fat: 7g; Sodium: 333mg; Protein: 7g; Fiber: 5g

1. Cover the mushrooms with the hot water, and set aside to soak for 10 minutes.

2. In a large skillet over medium heat, heat the oil. Add the shallot, garlic, and a pinch salt. Cook for 3 to 4 minutes, until softened.

3. With a slotted spoon, strain the mushrooms, reserving the soaking liquid. Strain the soaking liquid to remove any sediment.

4. Roughly chop the mushrooms. Add them to the skillet, along with the soaking liquid and kale.

5. Simmer for about 20 minutes, until the kale is very soft and the liquid has mostly evaporated.

continued ↪

6. Stir in the coconut milk, miso, soy sauce, and vinegar, and cook for 1 to 2 minutes to allow the flavors to come together and the sauce to thicken slightly.

7. Season with salt and pepper and serve.

SUBSTITUTION TIP: If you don't have dried shiitake mushrooms, you can use another dried wild mushroom. Fresh mushrooms can also be used, but they should be sliced and cooked in step 2 with the shallots and garlic; also, use 1 cup of vegetable broth in place of the mushroom soaking liquid.

ROASTED FENNEL, ONION, AND CARROTS

Allergen-Free, Egg-Free, Gluten-Free, Nut-Free, Vegan

SERVES 4

PREP TIME: 5 minutes COOK TIME: 35 to 40 minutes

Oven roasting is the gateway to loving vegetables. They're perfectly tender and caramelized, and their flavors mellow and become sweeter. You can skip the carrots with tops if you wish, but the carrot greens are really so pretty—and they make a brilliant pesto to top this dish (see Serving tip).

1 bunch scrubbed carrots, with tops

1 large fennel bulb, trimmed and cut into wedges

1 red onion, halved and cut into ½-inch-thick half circles

2 tablespoons canola oil or extra-virgin olive oil

1 tablespoon minced fresh thyme or rosemary leaves

Sea salt

Freshly ground black pepper

Per Serving Calories: 144; Total Carbohydrates: 19g; Sugar: 7g; Total Fat: 7g; Saturated Fat: 1g; Sodium: 174mg; Protein: 2g; Fiber: 6g

1. Preheat the oven to 425°F. Line a sheet pan with parchment paper.

2. Remove all but 1 inch of the carrot tops and reserve for another use. Cut the carrots in half lengthwise.

3. Spread out the fennel, onion, and carrots on the pan. Drizzle with the oil and season with the thyme, salt, and pepper. Toss gently to coat.

4. Roast for 35 to 40 minutes, or until the vegetables are tender and browned on the bottom.

SERVING TIP: To make a carrot-top pesto, in a food processor, combine 1 cup of roughly chopped carrot tops (avoid the tough ends of the stems), ½ cup of fresh basil, 2 garlic cloves, 2 tablespoons of olive oil, and 1 tablespoon of freshly squeezed lemon juice. Purée until mostly smooth. Season with salt and pepper. Drizzle the pesto over the cooked vegetables.

ROSEMARY ROASTED POTATOES

Allergen-Free, Egg-Free, Gluten-Free, Nut-Free, Vegan

SERVES 4

PREP TIME: 5 minutes   COOK TIME: 40 to 45 minutes

Roasted potatoes are my go-to side dish because they're easy and delicious, especially when tossed with some fresh herbs. Rosemary works well because it withstands the high heat of oven roasting and infuses the potatoes with flavor. The potatoes develop a nice golden-brown skin on the outside and become luxuriously creamy on the inside.

1½ pounds Yukon Gold potatoes, scrubbed

1 tablespoon minced fresh rosemary leaves

2 tablespoons extra-virgin olive oil

Sea salt

Freshly ground black pepper

Per Serving Calories: 180; Total Carbohydrates: 27g; Sugar: 2g; Total Fat: 7g; Saturated Fat: 1g; Sodium: 69mg; Protein: 3g; Fiber: 4g

1. Preheat the oven to 375°F. Line a sheet pan with parchment paper.

2. Cut the smaller potatoes in half and the larger ones into quarters. Spread them out on the pan.

3. Sprinkle the potatoes with the rosemary and drizzle with the oil. Toss gently to coat, then season liberally with salt and pepper.

4. Roast uncovered for 40 to 45 minutes, until the tops are lightly golden and the bottoms are nicely caramelized.

INGREDIENT TIP: If you cannot find Yukon Gold potatoes, choose another small yellow potato.

SCALLOPED POTATOES

Egg-Free, Make Gluten-Free, Vegan

SERVES 6

PREP TIME: 10 minutes   COOK TIME: 40 minutes

Creamy on the inside with a nice golden crust on the outside, these scalloped potatoes are comfort food to the max. Perfect for holiday gatherings or summer barbecues, they will win over even the toughest critic.

3 tablespoons dairy-free butter, such as Earth Balance Buttery Spread, divided

2 tablespoons all-purpose flour or gluten-free flour blend

2 cups chicken broth or vegetable broth

1 teaspoon minced garlic

1 teaspoon minced fresh thyme leaves

1 teaspoon sea salt

1½ cups Cashew Cream (page 22)

2 pounds baking potatoes, sliced paper-thin

¼ cup Plant-Based Parmesan (page 27, optional)

Per Serving Calories: 270; Total Carbohydrates: 29g; Sugar: 3g; Total Fat: 16g; Saturated Fat: 10g; Sodium: 637mg; Protein: 5g; Fiber: 5g

1. Preheat the oven to 375°F. Coat the interior of a 2-quart casserole dish with 1 tablespoon of dairy-free butter.

2. In a medium saucepan, melt the remaining 2 tablespoons of dairy-free butter. Add the flour, and whisk until thick and bubbling, about 1 minute. Pour in the broth, and whisk constantly until thickened.

3. Stir in the garlic, thyme, salt, and cashew cream.

4. Spread the potatoes in the casserole dish, and pour the sauce over the top, stirring just to distribute the sauce. Top with the plant-based Parmesan (if using).

5. Bake uncovered for 40 minutes, until the potatoes are tender and the top is browned and bubbling.

INGREDIENT TIP: I like to use starchy potatoes such as russets in this recipe, because their starch thickens the sauce as they cook.

MASHED POTATOES

Egg-Free, Vegetarian

SERVES 4

PREP TIME: 5 minutes   COOK TIME: 15 minutes

I love the texture and flavor of mashed potatoes with dairy-free sour cream. If you prefer to skip that step, simply use another ½ to 1 cup of almond milk.

2 ½ pounds Yukon Gold potatoes, peeled and quartered

8 ounces Dairy-Free Sour Cream (page 192) or store-bought

2 tablespoons dairy-free butter, such as Earth Balance Buttery Spread

½ to 1 cup Plain Nut Milk (page 20) made with almonds

2 tablespoons minced fresh chives (optional)

Per Serving Calories: 373; Total Carbohydrates: 49g; Sugar: 7g; Total Fat: 18g; Saturated Fat: 12g; Sodium: 226mg; Protein: 6g; Fiber: 7g

1. Put the potatoes in a large pot of salted water. Bring to a boil, and cook until the potatoes are fork-tender, about 15 minutes.

2. Drain the potatoes thoroughly. Stir in the dairy-free sour cream and dairy-free butter, and mash with a potato masher. While mashing, add enough almond milk to thin the potatoes to your desired consistency.

3. Serve garnished with the chives (if using).

   COOKING TIP: If you use a potato ricer, you do not need to peel the potatoes.

BOURBON MASHED SWEET POTATOES

Egg-Free, Gluten-Free, Make Allergen-Free, Make Nut-Free, Vegan

SERVES 6

PREP TIME: 10 minutes COOK TIME: 45 minutes

I tried these for the first time at Thanksgiving and wanted to skip dessert just so I could lick the casserole dish clean. They're that good! They're also much healthier than the traditional marshmallow-topped sweet potatoes that are ubiquitous around the holidays.

½ cup dairy-free butter, such as Earth Balance Buttery Spread, plus 1 tablespoon

2 pounds sweet potatoes

¼ cup bourbon

¼ cup brown sugar

½ teaspoon sea salt

1 cup pecan halves, toasted

Per Serving Calories: 499; Total Carbohydrates: 51g; Sugar: 7g; Total Fat: 30g; Saturated Fat: 6g; Sodium: 336mg; Protein: 4g; Fiber: 8g

1. Preheat the oven to 375°F. Coat the interior of a 2-quart casserole dish with 1 tablespoon of dairy-free butter.

2. Peel the sweet potatoes and dice into 1-inch pieces. In a steamer over simmering water, steam the potatoes for 20 minutes or until tender.

3. Once cooked, drain and transfer the potatoes to a large bowl. Add the bourbon, sugar, the ½ cup of the dairy-free butter, and salt. With a potato masher, mash until smooth.

4. Spread the mixture into the casserole dish, and top with the pecans. Bake uncovered for 25 minutes.

SUBSTITUTION TIP: To make this nut-free, simply omit the pecans and proceed as directed.

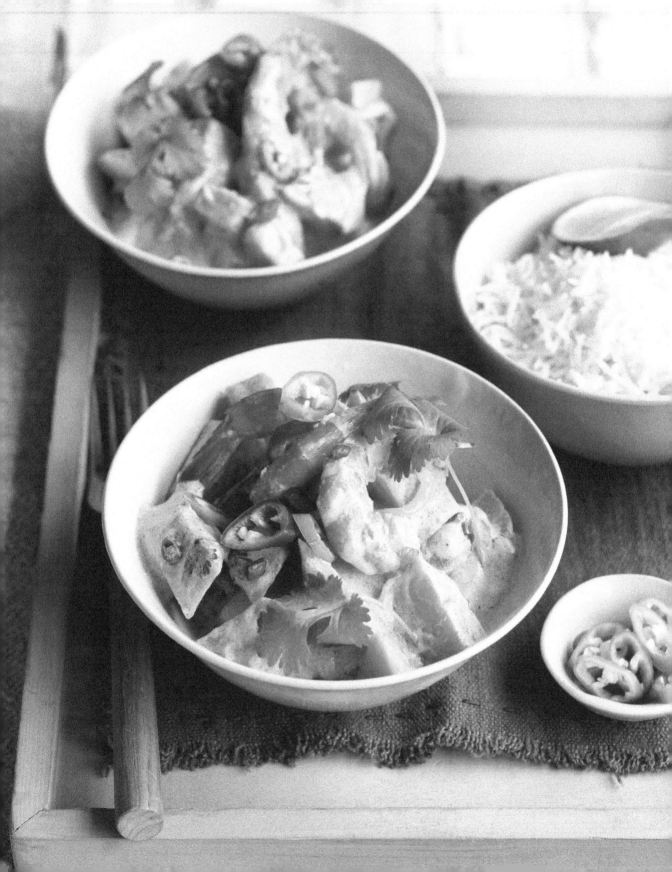

Chapter Seven

FISH AND SEAFOOD

CLAM CHOWDER

Egg-Free, Gluten-Free

SERVES 4

PREP TIME: 10 minutes COOK TIME: 45 minutes

Growing up in the Pacific Northwest, I knew that seafood was always on the menu, and I learned to like it from a young age, especially clam chowder. On dark days, a steaming bowl of chowder was the perfect antidote to a rained-out camping trip in the San Juan Islands or a drizzly hike through the Columbia Gorge.

4 bacon slices, roughly chopped

4 celery stalks, finely diced

1 onion, finely diced

4 garlic cloves, minced

Sea salt

8 ounces clam juice

1 thyme sprig

4 medium potatoes, peeled and diced

4 cups Plain Nut Milk (page 20) made with almonds, or Soy Milk (page 23), divided

2 (6-ounce) cans clams, drained and roughly chopped

Freshly ground black pepper

Per Serving Calories: 318; Total Carbohydrates: 40g; Sugar: 4g; Total Fat: 12g; Saturated Fat: 3g; Sodium: 885mg; Protein: 14g; Fiber: 7g

1. In a large pot over medium-low heat, cook the bacon for 10 minutes, until it has rendered most of its fat. Transfer the bacon to a separate dish, leaving the fat in the pot.

2. Add the celery, onion, and garlic to the pot and season with salt. Cook for 10 minutes.

3. Pour in the clam juice, add the thyme, and bring to a simmer. Add the potatoes, cover, and cook for 25 minutes, until tender. Remove and discard the thyme.

4. Remove about 1 cup of the potatoes, and in a blender, purée them with 1 cup of nut milk until smooth.

5. Return the purée to the pot along with the remaining 3 cups of nut or soy milk.

6. Bring to a gentle simmer, stir in the clams and bacon, and cook just until heated through.

7. Season with salt and pepper before serving.

SUBSTITUTION TIP: To make this soup without bacon, cook the vegetables in 2 tablespoons dairy-free butter. Add ¼ to ½ teaspoon liquid smoke when you add the clams.

SHRIMP BISQUE

Egg-Free, Make Gluten-Free, Make Nut-Free

SERVES 4

PREP TIME: 10 minutes COOK TIME: 30 minutes

Soup is one of my favorite meals to come home to after a long morning of surfing. Even in Santa Barbara, winter mornings spent in the water are chilly. This creamy seafood soup hits the spot. It is sweet and savory, and has just the right amount of kick from cayenne pepper. You can make it ahead of time; just wait to cook the shrimp and stir in the dairy-free cream until right before serving.

1½ pounds large shrimp

6 cups water

Sea salt

1 leek, halved and thoroughly cleaned

2 garlic cloves, smashed

2 celery stalks, roughly chopped

2 carrots, roughly chopped

¼ cup dairy-free butter, such as Earth Balance Buttery Spread

¼ cup all-purpose flour or gluten-free flour blend

Zest of 1 orange

2 tablespoons tomato paste

½ teaspoon cayenne pepper

1 cup dairy-free cream, such as Califia Dairy Free Better Half

Freshly ground black pepper

Per Serving Calories: 469; Total Carbohydrates: 35g; Sugar: 23g; Total Fat: 19g; Saturated Fat: 9g; Sodium: 604mg; Protein: 38g; Fiber: 2g

1. Peel the shrimp and place the peels in a large pot over medium heat. Cover with the water, a pinch salt, the leek, garlic, celery, and carrots. Bring to a simmer, and cook for 20 minutes.

2. Strain the broth, reserving it and discarding the shells and vegetables. Set the broth aside.

3. Wipe the pot clean, then cook the dairy-free butter and flour over medium heat for 1 to 2 minutes, whisking constantly until thick and bubbling.

4. Pour in the shrimp stock, whisking vigorously. Add the orange zest, tomato paste, and cayenne. Simmer for 5 minutes to thicken.

continued ☞

5. Add the shrimp, and simmer until cooked through, 2 to 3 minutes. Stir in the dairy-free cream, and cook until just heated through. Season with salt and pepper.

INGREDIENT TIP: My favorite gluten-free flour blend for thickening soups and sauces is Bob's Red Mill Gluten Free 1-to-1 Baking Flour. It is starchy and performs more like all-purpose flour than other brands.

INGREDIENT TIP: If you need to follow a nut-free diet, choose a dairy-free cream that doesn't contain nuts. The brand suggested in this recipe contains almond milk and coconut cream.

BUTTERNUT SQUASH AND SHRIMP CURRY

Egg-Free, Gluten-Free, Nut-Free

SERVES 4

PREP TIME: 10 minutes COOK TIME: 25 minutes

This Thai curry bowl is brimming with Southeast Asian flavors. Creamy coconut milk, pungent fish sauce, and fragrant lemongrass combine for an unforgettable and addicting broth. The butternut squash provides some carbs, but for an even more filling meal, serve with rice.

1 tablespoon coconut oil

1 red onion, halved and sliced

4 garlic cloves, minced

1 (1-inch) piece ginger, peeled and minced

1 Thai chile, minced

1 tablespoon minced lemongrass

1 tablespoon fish sauce

1 (15-ounce) can coconut milk

4 cups diced butternut squash (see Ingredient tip)

1½ pounds shrimp

1 tablespoon freshly squeezed lime juice

Sea salt

Freshly ground black pepper

½ cup fresh cilantro leaves

Per Serving Calories: 530; Total Carbohydrates: 28g; Sugar: 9g; Total Fat: 31g; Saturated Fat: 26g; Sodium: 811mg; Protein: 40g; Fiber: 6g

1. In a large pot over medium heat, heat the oil. Add the onion, garlic, ginger, and chile, and cook, stirring occasionally, until fragrant and nearly soft, about 5 minutes.

2. Add the lemongrass, fish sauce, and coconut milk. Bring to a simmer, and add the butternut squash. Cover and simmer until the butternut squash is tender, about 15 minutes.

3. Add the shrimp to the soup, and simmer for another 2 to 3 minutes, or until the shrimp are cooked through.

4. Stir in the lime juice, and season with salt and pepper.

5. Sprinkle with the cilantro before serving.

INGREDIENT TIP: To process the butternut squash, remove all of the peel with a vegetable peeler. Cut it in half lengthwise. Scoop out the seeds with a spoon. Cut the squash into 1-inch spears, and then cut into 1-inch dice.

COD WITH TOMATO-BASIL SAUCE

Egg-Free, Gluten-Free, Nut-Free

SERVES 4

PREP TIME: 5 minutes COOK TIME: 20 minutes

This easy one-pan supper has become my favorite recipe for cod, which can sometimes taste a little fishy. The spicy red pepper flakes, tangy tomatoes, lemon, and sweet basil are an addicting combination and pack a nice flavor punch for minimal effort. This dish is especially great in late summer, when tomatoes and basil are at their peak.

2 tablespoons extra-virgin olive oil

2 teaspoons minced garlic

Pinch red pepper flakes

2 pints grape tomatoes, halved

½ cup dry white wine

2 tablespoons freshly squeezed lemon juice

½ cup roughly chopped fresh basil, divided

4 (4- to 6-ounce) cod fillets

Sea salt

Freshly ground black pepper

Per Serving Calories: 258; Total Carbohydrates: 9g; Sugar: 5g; Total Fat: 9g; Saturated Fat: 1g; Sodium: 192mg; Protein: 32g; Fiber: 2g

1. In a large skillet over medium heat, heat the oil. Cook the garlic and red pepper flakes for 30 seconds, until fragrant.

2. Add the tomatoes, and cook for about 10 minutes, until thoroughly broken down.

3. Add the wine, and cook to burn off some of the alcohol. Add the lemon juice and ¼ cup of basil.

4. Season the cod fillets with salt and pepper. Place them in the skillet and top with some of the tomato–basil mixture. Simmer for 3 to 4 minutes, flip and then cook for another 3 to 4 minutes or until the fish flakes easily with a fork.

5. Garnish with the remaining ¼ cup of basil just before serving.

VARIATION TIP: For more Mediterranean flavors, use halibut and add 1 tablespoon minced fresh oregano and ½ cup whole green olives to the skillet.

MISO-GLAZED COD

Egg-Free, Nut-Free, Make Gluten-Free

SERVES 4

PREP TIME: 5 minutes COOK TIME: 15 to 20 minutes

This Asian-inspired baked cod is sweet and savory, with unexpected flavors that come from the mellow white miso paste. Double the sauce to add to some sautéed vegetables. Serve with steamed rice or buckwheat noodles.

2 tablespoons white miso paste

2 tablespoons low-sodium soy sauce

1 tablespoon rice vinegar

1 tablespoon toasted sesame oil

½ tablespoon honey

4 (4- to 6-ounce) cod fillets

2 tablespoons sesame seeds

Per Serving Calories: 220; Total Carbohydrates: 7g; Sugar: 3g; Total Fat: 7g; Saturated Fat: 1g; Sodium: 832mg; Protein: 32g; Fiber: 1g

1. Preheat the oven to 350°F.

2. In a small bowl, whisk together the miso, soy sauce, vinegar, oil, and honey.

3. Place the cod in a baking dish, and cover with the miso sauce, turning the fish to coat.

4. Cover and bake for 10 minutes. Remove the cover and bake for another 5 to 10 minutes, or until the cod is cooked through and flakes easily with a fork.

5. Meanwhile, toast the sesame seeds in a dry skillet until golden brown and fragrant. Sprinkle the toasted sesame seeds over the cod to serve.

INGREDIENT TIP: To make this dish gluten-free, use gluten-free soy sauce.

INGREDIENT TIP: Miso is fermented soybean paste with a salty, sweet, and complex flavor. Choose mellow white miso for this recipe.

SOLE MEUNIÈRE

Egg-Free, Gluten-Free, Nut-Free

SERVES 2

PREP TIME: 5 minutes COOK TIME: 5 minutes

I first enjoyed sole meunière in England after purchasing fresh fish from a fisherman in Aldeburgh, a small town on the North Sea. I was thrilled to discover that the classic French recipe—a highlight of Julia Child's early dining experiences in France—is a cinch to prepare. It is traditionally made with browned butter, however, the Maillard reaction also occurs using dairy-free butter, yielding that delicious browned taste.

¼ cup all-purpose flour or gluten-free flour blend

½ teaspoon fine sea salt

¼ teaspoon freshly ground black pepper

2 (10- to 14-ounce) whole sole fillets

2 tablespoons dairy-free butter, such as Earth Balance Buttery Spread

Juice of 1 lemon

1 tablespoon minced fresh parsley

Per Serving Calories: 508; Total Carbohydrates: 12g; Sugar: 0g; Total Fat: 18g; Saturated Fat: 3g; Sodium: 894mg; Protein: 75g; Fiber: 1g

1. In a shallow dish, mix together the flour, salt, and pepper. Pat the fish dry with paper towels, and dredge in the flour mixture.

2. In a wide skillet over medium-high heat, heat the dairy-free butter. Sear the fish on one side for about 2 minutes. Turn carefully and cook on the other side for 1 to 2 minutes or until just cooked through.

3. Transfer the fish to a serving platter.

4. Drizzle the lemon juice into the skillet, scraping up the browned bits, then pour over the cooked fish and sprinkle with the fresh parsley. Serve immediately.

SUBSTITUTION TIP: Sole is not always a sustainable seafood option, so you can use another flaky, flat white fish if you like.

CAJUN BLACKENED HALIBUT WITH SAUTÉED PEPPERS

Egg-Free, Gluten-Free, Nut-Free

SERVES 4

PREP TIME: 10 minutes COOK TIME: 15 minutes

Here, spicy blackened halibut joins with sautéed peppers and onions in a tangy pan sauce. While blackening might suggest the fish is burned, it is not. Blackening spices darken when cooked, but the fish remains perfectly moist. Serve this tasty dish with steamed rice.

2 tablespoons Cajun blackening spice

2 tablespoons minced fresh parsley

1 teaspoon minced fresh garlic

3 tablespoons canola oil, divided

½ teaspoon sea salt, plus more for seasoning

¼ teaspoon freshly ground black pepper, plus more for seasoning

4 (4- to 6-ounce) halibut fillets

1 red or yellow bell pepper, cored and thinly sliced

1 green bell pepper, cored and thinly sliced

½ yellow onion, thinly sliced

¼ cup white wine

1 tablespoon freshly squeezed lemon juice

Per Serving Calories: 303; Total Carbohydrates: 6g; Sugar: 3g; Total Fat: 15g; Saturated Fat: 1g; Sodium: 349mg; Protein: 36g; Fiber: 1g

1. With a mortar and pestle, crush the blackening spice, parsley, garlic, 2 tablespoons of oil, the salt, and pepper until it forms a paste. Spread the paste onto the fish, coating all sides.

2. Heat a large skillet over medium-high heat. Cook the fillets for 3 to 4 minutes on each side, until they are dark on the outside and flake easily with a fork. Transfer to a serving platter.

3. Add the remaining 1 tablespoon of oil to the skillet. Sauté the peppers and onion until just softened and beginning to brown, about 3 minutes.

4. Add the wine and lemon juice, and cook for 2 minutes. Season with salt and pepper. Serve alongside the fish.

COOKING TIP: For extra flavor, coat the fish in the spice paste up to 8 hours ahead of time and keep refrigerated until ready to cook.

STEAMED MUSSELS

Egg-Free, Gluten-Free, Nut-Free

SERVES 4

PREP TIME: 5 minutes COOK TIME: 20 minutes

These mussels are ubiquitous on appetizer menus and are perfect for serving with a simple side salad and a generous hunk of bread for dunking. You can also serve these over fresh pasta. Although clams are often prepared the same way, I prefer the tenderness of mussels.

4 tablespoons extra-virgin olive oil, divided

2 shallots, minced

4 garlic cloves, minced

½ cup dry white wine

½ cup chicken broth

4 thyme sprigs

2 pounds fresh mussels, scrubbed, debearded, and rinsed

Sea salt

Freshly ground black pepper

¼ cup fresh Italian parsley, roughly chopped

1 lemon, halved

Per Serving Calories: 354; Total Carbohydrates: 11g; Sugar: 0g; Total Fat: 19g; Saturated Fat: 3g; Sodium: 807mg; Protein: 28g; Fiber: 0g

1. In a large pot over medium heat, heat the oil. Add the shallots and garlic, and cook, stirring occasionally, until soft, about 5 minutes. Stir in the wine, chicken broth, thyme, and mussels.

2. Season with salt and pepper, give everything a good toss, cover, and allow the mussels to steam open, about 10 minutes.

3. Remove the cooked mussels to a bowl, discard any that did not open, and cover the bowl.

4. Continue simmering the cooking liquid until reduced by about half, about 5 minutes. Pour the liquid over the cooked mussels, garnish with the parsley, squeeze with lemon juice, and serve immediately.

INGREDIENT TIP: Scrub and debeard the mussels just before you intend to cook them. Discard any mussels that are broken or already open and don't close when tapped gently.

SPICY ITALIAN SAUSAGE AND MUSSELS OVER FETTUCINE

Egg-Free, Gluten-Free, Nut-Free

SERVES 4

PREP TIME: 5 minutes COOK TIME: 25 to 30 minutes

Is there anything more comforting than a giant shared platter of pasta topped with flavorful sausage, tomatoes, and fresh mussels? It's one of my favorite dishes for serving to company because we can enjoy it family-style, and dinner lasts a little longer because the mussels are still in their shells.

12 ounces fettucine

2 tablespoons olive oil

1 red onion, halved and thinly sliced

6 garlic cloves, smashed

2 spicy Italian sausage links, casings removed

1 cup dry white wine

½ cup chicken broth

2 tablespoons tomato paste

1 (15-ounce) can whole plum tomatoes, drained, crushed

½ cup hand-torn fresh basil leaves

2 pounds fresh mussels, scrubbed and debearded

Per Serving Calories: 616; Total Carbohydrates: 68g; Sugar: 6g; Total Fat: 15g; Saturated Fat: 3g; Sodium: 909mg; Protein: 42g; Fiber: 13g

1. Bring a large pot of salted water to a boil, and cook the pasta according to the package directions, about 10 minutes. Drain the pasta and set aside.

2. While the pasta cooks, in a large pot over medium heat, heat the oil. Add the onion and garlic, and cook for 3 to 4 minutes, stirring occasionally, until beginning to soften.

3. Add the sausage, and cook for 2 to 3 minutes.

4. Add the wine, chicken broth, tomato paste, and tomatoes, and bring to a simmer. Cook uncovered for 10 minutes.

5. Add the basil and mussels to the pot, give everything a good toss, cover, and cook until the mussels have steamed open, up to 10 minutes. Discard any that did not open.

6. Place the pasta in a large serving dish, and pour the sausage, mussels, and broth over the pasta. Give everything a good toss before serving.

INGREDIENT TIP: If you want a little more spice than the Italian sausage brings to the party, add a generous pinch red pepper flakes.

SEARED GARLIC SCALLOPS AND LINGUINE

Egg-Free, Gluten-Free, Nut-Free

SERVES 4

PREP TIME: 5 minutes COOK TIME: 15 minutes

Fresh sea scallops cooked with garlic, parsley, and fresh lemon juice is a simple and delicious combination atop a bed of linguine. Use fresh pasta for an extra special meal. Whether you use fresh or dried pasta, the starches from the pasta cooking liquid create a thick, creamy pan sauce without using a drop of cream.

12 ounces linguine

2 tablespoons canola oil

1 pound large sea scallops

Sea salt

Freshly ground black pepper

1 tablespoon minced garlic

¼ cup minced fresh parsley

2 tablespoons freshly squeezed lemon juice

Per Serving Calories: 485; Total Carbohydrates: 68g; Sugar: 3g; Total Fat: 9g; Saturated Fat: 1g; Sodium: 250mg; Protein: 31g; Fiber: 3g

1. Bring a large pot of salted water to a boil. Cook the pasta according to the package directions, about 10 minutes. Drain the pasta, reserving ⅓ cup of the cooking liquid.

2. Heat a large skillet over high heat until very hot. Add the oil, and tilt to coat the bottom. Allow the oil to heat for 30 seconds.

3. Pat the scallops dry with paper towels, and season generously with salt and pepper.

4. Sear the scallops for 2 minutes on one side, basting them with the pan juices.

5. Flip the scallops, and sear on the other side for 2 minutes.

6. During the last minute of cooking, add the garlic, parsley, and lemon juice to the pan, continuing to baste the scallops with the pan juices.

7. Add the pasta to the pan, along with the reserved pasta cooking liquid. Give everything a good toss, season with salt and pepper, and divide between serving plates.

COOKING TIP: To baste the scallops, tilt the pan slightly, and use a spoon to scoop up the pan juices and drizzle them over the scallops.

FISH TACOS WITH CILANTRO-LIME CREMA

Egg-Free, Gluten-Free, Nut-Free

SERVES 4

PREP TIME: 10 minutes COOK TIME: 5 minutes

Restaurant-quality fish tacos are easy to make at home, but what really makes these shine is the homemade cilantro crema. Dairy-free sour cream and mayonnaise are blended with fresh cilantro, lime, and jalapeño for a spicy, tangy sauce.

For the fish

2 tablespoons canola oil

1 teaspoon ground cumin

1 teaspoon smoked paprika

1 teaspoon dried oregano

½ teaspoon sea salt

½ teaspoon freshly ground black pepper

1 pound mahi-mahi, swordfish, or other firm white fish

For the cilantro-lime crema

½ cup mayonnaise

½ cup Dairy-Free Sour Cream (page 192) or store-bought

Zest and juice of 1 lime

½ cup roughly chopped fresh cilantro

½ small jalapeño pepper, seeded

For serving

8 corn tortillas

1 cup pico de gallo salsa

1 cup shredded cabbage

Per Serving Calories: 412; Total Carbohydrates: 31g; Sugar: 5g; Total Fat: 21g; Saturated Fat: 10g; Sodium: 795mg; Protein: 27g; Fiber: 5g

To make the fish

1. In a small dish, mix the oil, cumin, paprika, oregano, salt, and pepper. Add the mahi-mahi and toss gently to coat in the marinade.

2. Preheat a grill pan to medium-high. Cook the mahi-mahi for 4 to 5 minutes, turning as needed until just cooked through. Break into bite-size pieces.

To make the cilantro-lime crema

In a blender, combine all the ingredients. Purée until smooth.

To assemble the tacos

To serve, top each corn tortilla with a few pieces of mahi-mahi, a scoop of pico de gallo, a pinch shredded cabbage, and a generous drizzle of cilantro-lime crema.

COOKING TIP: I use an immersion blender when mixing smaller amounts of ingredients, but a regular countertop blender will also work.

CRAB CAKES WITH LEMON AIOLI

Make Gluten-Free, Nut-Free

SERVES 4

PREP TIME: 10 minutes   COOK TIME: 10 minutes

Crab is a classic, but pretty much any seafood can be used in these simple crab cakes. As with the Fish Tacos with Cilantro-Lime Crema (page 99), the sauce really does make the dish here. Instead of using a dairy-free sour cream, however, this version is made with prepared mayonnaise spiked with fresh lemon juice. It is tangy and delicious.

2 scallions, thinly sliced

2 garlic cloves, minced, plus 1 teaspoon minced

1 pound lump crab meat, picked over for shells

1 cup fresh bread crumbs

1 egg white

¼ teaspoon Old Bay seasoning

¼ teaspoon sea salt

¼ teaspoon freshly ground black pepper

⅓ cup mayonnaise

2 tablespoons freshly squeezed lemon juice

2 tablespoons canola oil

Leaves of 1 mint sprig, roughly chopped

Per Serving Calories: 338; Total Carbohydrates: 27g; Sugar: 3g; Total Fat: 24g; Saturated Fat: 2g; Sodium: 1105mg; Protein: 21g; Fiber: 2g

1. In a small bowl, mix the scallions, 2 minced garlic cloves, crab meat, bread crumbs, egg white, Old Bay seasoning, salt, and pepper. Form the mixture into 8 cakes. Set aside to firm up and allow the flavors to come together.

2. In a small bowl, whisk together the mayonnaise, lemon juice, and 1 teaspoon of minced garlic. Cover and refrigerate until ready to serve.

3. Heat a large skillet over medium-high heat. Add the oil, and fry the crab cakes for 4 to 5 minutes on each side, until a golden crust forms.

4. To serve, drizzle with the lemon aioli and garnish with the mint.

SUBSTITUTION TIP: Use gluten-free bread to make this recipe gluten-free.

CORIANDER-CRUSTED SALMON OVER ARUGULA

Egg-Free, Gluten-Free, Nut-Free

SERVES 4

PREP TIME: 5 minutes COOK TIME: 5 to 6 minutes

Ground coriander and black pepper make a delicious crust for fresh salmon. The recipe is naturally dairy-free and is complemented by peppery fresh arugula. Serve with roasted potatoes for a complete meal.

1 tablespoon whole coriander seeds

1 teaspoon peppercorns

½ teaspoon sea salt, plus more for seasoning

4 (4- to 6-ounce) salmon fillets

2 tablespoons extra-virgin olive oil, divided

1 tablespoon freshly squeezed lemon juice

1 teaspoon Dijon mustard

1 teaspoon honey

Freshly ground black pepper

4 cups fresh arugula

Per Serving Calories: 473; Total Carbohydrates: 3g; Sugar: 2g; Total Fat: 27g; Saturated Fat: 5g; Sodium: 365mg; Protein: 49g; Fiber: 1g

1. Grind the coriander and peppercorns in a spice grinder or mortar and pestle. Add the salt to the spices, and stir to mix.

2. Pat the spice mixture onto the salmon. You can do this up to 8 hours ahead of time.

3. Heat a large skillet over medium-high heat. Add 1 tablespoon of oil to the skillet and tilt to coat the bottom.

4. Sear the salmon for 2½ to 3 minutes on each side, until a nice brown crust forms and the salmon is nearly cooked through.

5. In a mixing bowl, whisk the remaining 1 tablespoon of oil with the lemon juice, mustard, and honey. Season with salt and pepper. Add the arugula and toss to coat. Divide the arugula between serving platters and top with the salmon.

COOKING TIP: The key with salmon is to not overcook it. It should still be a darker shade of pink when removed from the heat, as residual heat in the fish will cook it a bit more.

ROSEMARY-SEARED TUNA

Egg-Free, Gluten-Free, Nut-Free

SERVES 4

PREP TIME: 5 minutes COOK TIME: 2 to 3 minutes

Fresh seafood abounds in Santa Barbara, California, where I live. On Saturday mornings, there is a fish market at the harbor. Fortunately, the fresh flavors of the ocean are becoming easier to come by inland. If you don't have a fish market nearby, flash-frozen ahi tuna steaks work splendidly in this recipe. Defrost in the refrigerator the day you intend to cook them.

4 (4- to 6-ounce) ahi tuna steaks

1 tablespoon minced fresh rosemary leaves

Sea salt

Freshly ground black pepper

1 tablespoon canola oil

Per Serving Calories: 220; Total Carbohydrates: 1g; Sugar: 0g; Total Fat: 4g; Saturated Fat: 0g; Sodium: 135mg; Protein: 42g; Fiber: 0g

1. Heat a large skillet over high heat until very hot.

2. Pat the tuna dry with paper towels and season with the rosemary, salt, and pepper.

3. Add the oil to the skillet, and tilt to coat the bottom. Sear the tuna for 60 seconds on each side for rare, 90 seconds for medium-rare. The center should still be deep pink.

4. Serve immediately.

   SERVING TIP: Serve with Roasted Sweet Potato Salad (page 56).

TUNA CASSEROLE

Make Gluten-Free

SERVES 4

PREP TIME: 10 minutes COOK TIME: 35 to 40 minutes

Creamy, comforting casseroles can still be part of a dairy-free diet. This version is made with chicken broth, almond milk, and dairy-free butter. A splash of the noodles' cooking liquid further thickens the sauce. It's also lighter in calories than the traditional version, but still loaded with flavor.

3 tablespoons dairy-free butter, such as Earth Balance Buttery Spread, divided

12 ounces egg noodles or gluten-free pasta

1 cup minced onion

¼ cup minced celery

2 tablespoons all-purpose flour or gluten-free flour blend

1 cup chicken broth

1 cup Plain Nut Milk (page 20) made with almonds or cashews

1 cup frozen peas, thawed

2 (5-ounce) cans tuna, drained

Sea salt

Freshly ground black pepper

1 cup wheat or gluten-free bread crumbs

Per Serving Calories: 546; Total Carbohydrates: 74g; Sugar: 6g; Total Fat: 13g; Saturated Fat: 3g; Sodium: 535mg; Protein: 33g; Fiber: 6g

1. Preheat the oven to 350°F. Coat the interior of a 2-quart casserole dish with 1 tablespoon of dairy-free butter.

2. Bring a large pot of salted water to a boil. Cook the egg noodles according to the package directions, about 10 minutes. Drain the noodles, reserving ½ cup of the cooking liquid.

3. In a large pot over medium heat, melt the remaining 2 tablespoons of dairy-free butter. Add the onion and celery, and cook until soft, 5 to 7 minutes.

4. Stir in the flour, and cook for 1 minute.

5. Pour in the chicken broth and nut milk, and bring to a simmer. Cook, stirring occasionally, until thick and bubbling, 2 to 3 minutes. Stir in the noodles' cooking liquid.

6. Fold in the peas, tuna, and cooked pasta. Season with salt and pepper.

7. Spread the noodles into the prepared casserole dish. Top with the bread crumbs. Bake for 15 to 17 minutes, until the top is golden brown.

INGREDIENT TIP: Choose solid albacore tuna, which has larger pieces and a mild flavor perfect for this recipe.

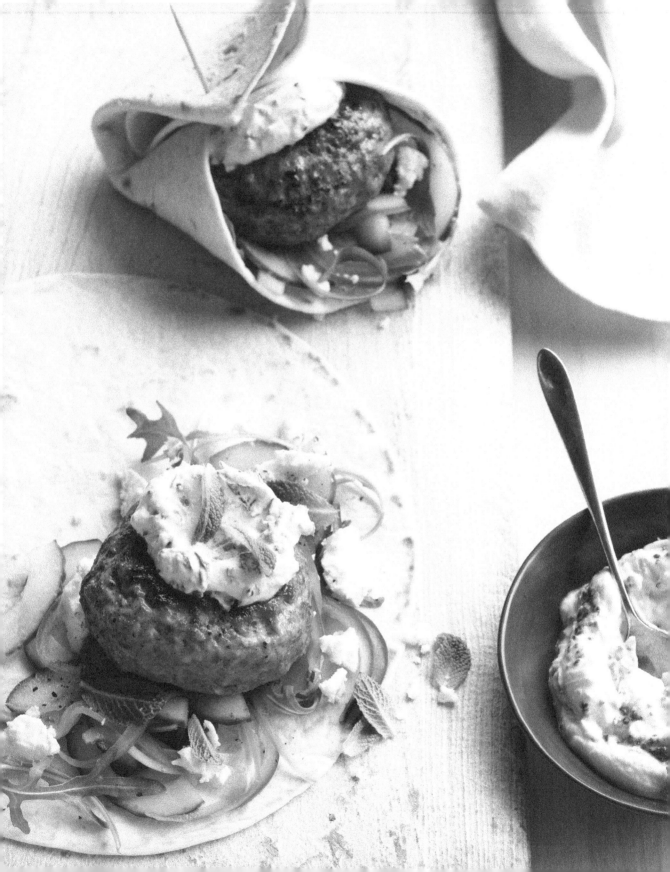

Chapter Eight

PORK AND BEEF

PEPPERONI, RED ONION, AND CHERRY TOMATO PIZZA

Make Gluten-Free, Make Egg-Free, Nut-Free, Make Allergen-Free

SERVES 4

PREP TIME: 10 minutes COOK TIME: 10 to 12 minutes

Combining Tofu Ricotta with dairy-free mozzarella makes this pie especially creamy and delicious. Pepperoni, onion, tomatoes, and fresh herbs are a simple but winning flavor combination. I like using a cast iron skillet and fresh pizza dough for a deep-dish option—just remember to par-bake the crust for 10 minutes before proceeding with the recipe. Enjoy it with a nice bottle of red wine.

1 (12-inch) prepared pizza crust

1 cup Pomodoro Sauce (page 195) or store-bought marinara sauce

2 tablespoons minced fresh herbs, such as basil and oregano

1 cup Tofu Ricotta (page 29)

1 cup shredded dairy-free mozzarella such as Follow Your Heart

16 slices good-quality pepperoni

1 small red onion, halved and thinly sliced

¼ cup black olives, such as Kalamata

½ cup halved cherry tomatoes

Per Serving Calories: 411; Total Carbohydrates: 30g; Sugar: 10g; Total Fat: 28g; Saturated Fat: 12g; Sodium: 1361mg; Protein: 12g; Fiber: 5g

1. Preheat the oven to 400°F.

2. Place the pizza crust on a large pan and spread the sauce over the crust. Sprinkle with the fresh herbs.

3. Drop the tofu ricotta by the tablespoon over the entire pizza, and top with the dairy-free mozzarella.

4. Layer the pepperoni, onion, olives, and cherry tomatoes on the pizza.

5. Bake for 10 to 12 minutes, until the sauce is hot and bubbling and the crust begins to brown.

SUBSTITUTION TIP: To make this gluten- and allergen-free, use a gluten-free pizza crust made without eggs.

CARNITAS TACOS

Allergen-Free, Egg-Free, Gluten-Free, Nut-Free

SERVES 6

PREP TIME: 10 minutes COOK TIME: 2 hours 15 minutes

My kids' school is predominantly Hispanic, so when holidays roll around, the customary bake sale items are upstaged by the most amazing Mexican food—carnitas, barbacoa, tamales—it's all so delicious! Carnitas tacos are one of my favorites. Although this recipe takes a long time to cook, only 15 minutes of it is active time.

1 (1½-pound) boneless pork shoulder

Sea salt

Freshly ground black pepper

2 tablespoons canola oil

1 tablespoon ground cumin

2 teaspoons dried oregano

1¼ teaspoons ground cinnamon

1 teaspoon ground coriander

⅛ teaspoon ground cloves

Zest and juice of 1 orange

1 red onion, halved and sliced

4 garlic cloves, roughly chopped

2 cups chicken broth

12 corn tortillas

1 bunch radishes, thinly sliced

2 cups shredded green cabbage

1 avocado, sliced

2 limes, cut into wedges, for serving

Per Serving Calories: 543; Total Carbohydrates: 30g; Sugar: 3g; Total Fat: 36g; Saturated Fat: 10g; Sodium: 376mg; Protein: 25g; Fiber: 7g

1. Preheat the oven to 325°F.

2. Cut the pork into 1-inch chunks. Season on all sides with salt and pepper.

3. Heat the oil in a Dutch oven or large oven-safe skillet with a lid over medium-high heat. Sear the pork on all sides until well browned, 10 to 15 minutes.

4. Add the cumin, oregano, cinnamon, coriander, cloves, orange zest and juice, onion, garlic, and chicken broth. Bring to a simmer.

5. Cover the Dutch oven and transfer to the oven. Roast for 2 hours, until the pork is tender. Shred the meat with a fork and serve in the corn tortillas. Top with radish slices, cabbage, and avocado, and serve with lime wedges.

COOKING TIP: To make this in a slow cooker, sear the meat and then transfer it to a slow cooker along with the spices, onion, garlic, and broth. Cover and cook on low for 8 to 10 hours or on high for 4 to 6 hours.

CREAMY TOMATO AND SAUSAGE PENNE

Egg-Free, Gluten-Free, Nut-Free

SERVES 4

PREP TIME: 5 minutes **COOK TIME:** 25 minutes

The first time I used pasta made from red lentil flour, I was amazed at its ability to create a rich, creamy sauce that bound the entire dish together. It is gluten-free and packed with protein!

8 ounces spicy Italian sausage, casings removed

1 red onion, diced

4 garlic cloves, roughly chopped

1 (15-ounce) can plum tomatoes, hand crushed

4 cups chicken broth

12 ounces red lentil penne pasta

½ cup roughly chopped fresh basil

¼ cup Plant-Based Parmesan (page 27), for serving

Per Serving Calories: 488; Total Carbohydrates: 67g; Sugar: 8g; Total Fat: 10g; Saturated Fat: 2g; Sodium: 1118mg; Protein: 32g; Fiber: 8g

1. Heat a large pot over medium-high heat. Cook the sausage for 2 to 3 minutes, until it renders some of its fat but is not yet cooked through.

2. Add the onion and garlic, and sauté for 1 to 2 minutes.

3. Add the tomatoes, chicken broth, and pasta, and bring to a simmer. Cover and cook for 20 minutes.

4. Stir in the basil, and allow the dish to rest for a few minutes to thicken before serving. Sprinkle with the plant-based Parmesan.

INGREDIENT TIP: Red lentil penne pasta is available at Trader Joe's, Whole Foods, and other healthy grocery stores, as well as online.

COCONUT-GINGER PORK TENDERLOIN SKEWERS

Allergen-Free, Egg-Free, Gluten-Free, Nut-Free

SERVES 4

PREP TIME: 5 minutes, plus at least 15 minutes to marinate COOK TIME: 15 minutes

Creamy coconut milk, fragrant ginger, and pungent spices marry beautifully in this marinade for pork tenderloin. It can be prepared in the oven or outside over a grill. This dish makes for excellent leftovers, so whip up a double batch!

½ cup coconut milk

2 tablespoons peeled and roughly chopped ginger

1 shallot, roughly chopped

1 tablespoon brown sugar

2 teaspoons ground coriander

½ teaspoon ground cumin

¼ teaspoon ground cayenne pepper

1 teaspoon sea salt

1 (1½-pound) pork tenderloin, cut into 2-inch pieces

Per Serving Calories: 279; Total Carbohydrates: 5g; Sugar: 3g; Total Fat: 15g; Saturated Fat: 8g; Sodium: 594mg; Protein: 37g; Fiber: 1g

1. Preheat the oven to 400°F. Line a sheet pan with parchment paper.

2. In a blender, combine the coconut milk, ginger, shallot, brown sugar, coriander, cumin, cayenne, and salt. Purée until smooth.

3. Pour the marinade over the pork tenderloin, and allow to rest for at least 15 minutes, or up to 8 hours in the refrigerator.

4. Thread the pork onto skewers, and transfer to the sheet pan. Bake for 15 minutes or until cooked through but still tender.

SERVING TIP: These skewers are delicious over an herb salad. Toss together ½ cup each of mint leaves, roughly chopped basil, and roughly chopped cilantro with 4 cups of torn butter lettuce leaves. Make a quick vinaigrette with 2 tablespoons of freshly squeezed lime juice, 2 tablespoons of canola oil, and 1 teaspoon of honey. Season with salt and pepper, and toss gently to coat.

ROSEMARY PORK TENDERLOIN WITH PLUM SAUCE

Egg-Free, Gluten-Free, Make Allergen-Free, Nut-Free

SERVES 4

PREP TIME: 5 minutes   COOK TIME: 25 minutes

This pork tenderloin has everything going for it, as just a handful of ingredients come together to create a flavorful, restaurant-quality entrée. Serve with Mashed Potatoes (page 84) for a complete meal.

2 tablespoons canola oil

1 (1¼-pound) pork tenderloin

1 tablespoon minced fresh rosemary leaves

Sea salt

Freshly ground black pepper

½ red onion, halved and cut in thick half circles

1 cup dry red wine

½ cup plum sauce

Per Serving Calories: 389; Total Carbohydrates: 31g; Sugar: 25g; Total Fat: 10g; Saturated Fat: 2g; Sodium: 447mg; Protein: 30g; Fiber: 1g

1. Preheat the oven to 400°F.

2. Heat a large oven-safe skillet over medium-high heat. When hot, pour in the oil.

3. Pat the pork tenderloin dry with paper towels. Coat the pork in the rosemary and season generously with salt and pepper.

4. In the skillet, sear the pork on all sides until nicely browned, about 5 minutes total.

5. Add the onion to the skillet and transfer it to the oven. Cook for 10 to 15 minutes, until the pork reaches an internal temperature of 145°F.

6. Transfer the pork to a cutting board to rest.

7. Carefully return the pan to the stove top, and turn the heat to medium. Add the wine, and simmer until reduced to ½ cup, about 5 minutes. Stir in the plum sauce, and cook for 1 minute.

8. Slice the pork on a bias into ½-inch-thick medallions. Place them on a serving platter, and drizzle the plum sauce over the top.

INGREDIENT TIP: You can find plum sauce in the Asian section of the grocery store. It is sweet and tangy with a hint of spice. If you have allergies, read the label, as some varieties contain soy or wheat.

PORK MARSALA

Egg-Free, Make Allergen-Free, Make Gluten-Free, Nut-Free

SERVES 4

PREP TIME: 10 minutes COOK TIME: 20 minutes

The creamy, comforting flavors of pork marsala usually come from butter and flour. This version opts for neutral-flavored canola oil to brown the meat, and all-purpose or gluten-free flour can be used for thickening. Use a good-quality chicken broth, or make your own from roasted chicken bones for this recipe; its flavor really makes the sauce. See the Cooking tip for a quick roasted chicken stock.

3 tablespoons canola oil, divided

4 boneless pork loin chops, pounded to about ½-inch thickness

Sea salt

Freshly ground black pepper

2 tablespoons all-purpose flour or gluten-free flour blend

2 cups sliced mushrooms

½ yellow onion, minced

1 garlic clove, minced

1 teaspoon minced fresh thyme leaves

½ cup Marsala wine

½ cup chicken broth

Per Serving Calories: 339; Total Carbohydrates: 8g; Sugar: 2g; Total Fat: 22g; Saturated Fat: 5g; Sodium: 581mg; Protein: 23g; Fiber: 1g

1. Heat a large skillet over medium-high heat until hot. Add 2 tablespoons of oil, and tilt to coat the bottom.

2. Pat the pork dry with a paper towel, and season with salt and pepper. Sprinkle the chops lightly with the flour, shaking off any excess.

3. Place the pork in the skillet, and cook on each side for 3 minutes. Set aside.

4. Add the remaining 1 tablespoon of oil to the skillet, and sauté the mushrooms until browned, about 4 minutes.

continued ☞

5. Add the onion, garlic, and thyme to the pan, and cook for 30 seconds. Deglaze the pan with the wine, scraping up the browned bits. Add the chicken broth, and bring to a simmer.

6. Return the pork chops to the pan, cover, and finish cooking for 10 minutes.

COOKING TIP: To make your own chicken stock, roast 1 pound of chicken bones in a 400°F oven until deeply browned, about 30 minutes. Transfer the bones to a large pot, cover with 8 cups of water and a generous pinch sea salt, and simmer uncovered for 1½ to 2 hours, until the stock reaches your desired level of flavor and is reduced by about half. Strain the stock, discard the bones, and cool the liquid before covering and storing. It will keep for up to 5 days in the refrigerator or 3 months in the freezer.

RUSTIC ITALIAN MEATBALLS

Make Gluten-Free, Nut-Free

SERVES 4

PREP TIME: 10 minutes COOK TIME: 30 minutes

Parmesan and milk are often used in the commercially prepared meatballs that you would order in a restaurant or snag from the freezer section of the grocery store. Fortunately, soy milk or another dairy-free milk stands in easily for dairy, and fresh herbs and spices bring plenty of flavor to these meatballs.

2 slices white or gluten-free bread, torn into pieces

½ cup unsweetened, plain Soy Milk (page 23) or store-bought

1 small yellow onion, minced

4 garlic cloves, minced

1 egg, whisked

2 tablespoons minced fresh parsley

1 teaspoon minced fresh thyme leaves

1 teaspoon minced fresh oregano

1 teaspoon ground fennel seed

1 teaspoon sea salt

½ teaspoon freshly ground black pepper

⅛ teaspoon red pepper flakes

¾ pound ground beef

¾ pound ground pork

2 tablespoons extra-virgin olive oil

3 cups Pomodoro Sauce (page 195) or good-quality store-bought marinara sauce

¼ cup finely sliced fresh basil, for serving

½ cup Plant-Based Parmesan (page 27), for serving (optional)

Per Serving Calories: 528; Total Carbohydrates: 12g; Sugar: 5g; Total Fat: 42g; Saturated Fat: 14g; Sodium: 893mg; Protein: 26g; Fiber: 2g

1. Preheat the oven to 425°F.

2. Soak the bread in the soy milk for 1 minute. Remove it and squeeze out most of the excess moisture.

3. In a large bowl, mix together the soaked bread, onion, garlic, egg, parsley, thyme, oregano, fennel, salt, pepper, and red pepper flakes.

4. Add the beef and pork to the bowl, and use your hands to thoroughly mix. Shape the mixture into 8 to 12 large balls.

5. Heat a large oven-safe skillet over medium-high heat. Pour the oil into the skillet.

6. Fry the meatballs in the skillet, gently browning on all sides, for about 10 minutes.

continued ☞

7. Pour in the sauce, and transfer the skillet to the oven to bake for 15 to 18 minutes, until the sauce is bubbling and the meatballs are cooked through and tender.

8. Top with the basil and plant-based Parmesan (if using).

COOKING TIP: Typically, meatball recipes call for precooking the onion and garlic. This one saves that step, but cut the onion very finely so you don't find spicy, raw chunks of onion in the meatballs.

SWEDISH MEATBALLS

Make Gluten-Free, Nut-Free

SERVES 4

PREP TIME: 10 minutes COOK TIME: 30 to 35 minutes

Every time I wrap up my IKEA shopping trips, I pass the frozen case where the Swedish meatballs tempt me. Unfortunately, they contain dairy and beyond that, their ingredients have come under scrutiny, a good reminder that when you make things from scratch, you control the ingredients. And with this version, I can eliminate dairy but keep the creamy, comforting spice of the original.

2 slices white or gluten-free bread, torn into pieces

½ cup unsweetened, plain Soy Milk (page 23) or store-bought

2 tablespoons canola oil, divided

1 small yellow onion, minced

2 garlic cloves, minced

1 pound ground pork

½ pound ground beef

1 egg, whisked

½ teaspoon sea salt

¼ teaspoon ground allspice

¼ teaspoon ground nutmeg

2 tablespoons all-purpose flour or gluten-free flour blend

2 cups beef broth

¼ cup store-bought coconut cream

Per Serving Calories: 589; Total Carbohydrates: 14g; Sugar: 3g; Total Fat: 43g; Saturated Fat: 16g; Sodium: 832mg; Protein: 35g; Fiber: 2g

1. Preheat the oven to 200°F. Place a large baking dish in the oven to warm.

2. Soak the bread in the soy milk for 1 minute. Remove it and squeeze out most of the excess moisture.

3. Heat a large skillet over medium heat, and add 1 tablespoon of oil. Cook the onion and garlic until soft, 5 to 7 minutes.

4. In a large bowl, mix together the soaked bread, pork, beef, egg, salt, allspice, nutmeg, and the cooked onion and garlic until just integrated.

5. Form the meat mixture into 16 meatballs.

6. Add the remaining 1 tablespoon of oil to the skillet, and fry the meatballs until well browned on all sides and cooked through, 15 to 20 minutes. Transfer the meatballs to the warmed baking dish.

7. Return the skillet to the heat, and add the flour. Cook, stirring, until the flour soaks up the fat and begins to bubble, about 1 minute.

continued ☞

8. Add the beef broth and bring to a simmer, whisking constantly, until thickened, 2 to 3 minutes. Stir in the coconut cream until fully combined.

9. Return the meatballs to the skillet, and simmer for just 1 minute more.

COOKING TIP: Making meatballs is best done with your hands, but make sure to let the cooked onion mixture cool before handling it.

MEATBALL WRAPS WITH TZATZIKI

Make Gluten-Free, Nut-Free

SERVES 4

PREP TIME: 10 minutes COOK TIME: 20 minutes

Tzatziki, with its cooling mint and cucumber, provides the perfect complement to the full flavor of these lamb meatballs wrapped in soft flour tortillas. If you cannot find ground lamb, ground beef is a reasonable substitute.

1 plum tomato, finely diced

½ cup minced red onion

1 tablespoon minced garlic

1 egg, whisked

2 tablespoons minced fresh parsley

1 tablespoon minced fresh oregano

1 teaspoon sea salt

½ teaspoon freshly ground black pepper

1½ pounds ground lamb

4 flour tortillas

½ red onion, thinly sliced

½ cucumber, thinly sliced

1 cup arugula

¼ cup fresh mint leaves

1 cup Tzatziki (page 196)

Per Serving Calories: 603; Total Carbohydrates: 19g; Sugar: 5g; Total Fat: 47g; Saturated Fat: 18g; Sodium: 959mg; Protein: 29g; Fiber: 2g

1. Preheat the oven to 400°F.

2. In a large bowl, combine the tomato, onion, garlic, egg, parsley, oregano, salt, and pepper. Stir to mix.

3. Add the lamb, and use your hands to thoroughly mix. Shape the mixture into 8 meatballs.

4. Place the meatballs on a rimmed sheet pan, and bake for 20 minutes, or until lightly browned and cooked through.

5. To serve, place 2 meatballs on each tortilla, and top with the onion, cucumber, arugula, mint, and a generous spoonful of tzatziki sauce.

VARIATION TIP: Use butter lettuce leaves instead of tortillas for a low-carb, gluten-free option.

SHEPHERD'S PIE

Egg-Free, Gluten-Free, Make Allergen-Free, Make Nut-Free

SERVES 4

PREP TIME: 10 minutes COOK TIME: 35 minutes

My favorite dinners are the ones I can prepare ahead of time, leave in the refrigerator, and then simply pop into the oven at the end of a long day. This comforting shepherd's pie contains all of the classic ingredients of the original, with just a few minor tweaks to make it dairy-free.

2 tablespoons canola oil

1 yellow onion, diced

2 carrots, diced

1 cup finely chopped mushrooms

1 celery stalk, minced

2 garlic cloves, minced

1½ pounds ground beef or lamb

1 teaspoon minced fresh thyme leaves

1 teaspoon minced fresh rosemary leaves

1 cup frozen peas, thawed

1 tablespoon tomato paste

½ teaspoon sea salt, plus more for seasoning

Freshly ground black pepper

2 cups water

4 tablespoons dairy-free butter, such as Earth Balance Buttery Spread, divided

2 cups instant mashed potato flakes

1 cup Plain Nut Milk (page 20) or store-bought

Per Serving Calories: 563; Total Carbohydrates: 34g; Sugar: 6g; Total Fat: 31g; Saturated Fat: 8g; Sodium: 601mg; Protein: 39g; Fiber: 6g

1. Preheat the oven to 425°F.

2. In a large oven-safe skillet over medium heat, heat the oil. Cook the onion, carrots, mushrooms, celery, and garlic until soft and fragrant, about 10 minutes.

3. Push the vegetables to the side and add the beef, thyme, and rosemary to the skillet. Cook until the beef is just cooked through, about 10 minutes. Stir in the peas and tomato paste, and season generously with salt and pepper.

4. While the beef cooks, heat the water, ½ teaspoon of salt, and 3 tablespoons of dairy-free butter in a medium pot. Bring to a simmer and then stir in the potato flakes and nut milk. Stir until just combined.

5. Spread the mashed potatoes over the beef and vegetables. Melt the remaining 1 tablespoon of dairy-free butter and brush the top of the potatoes with it.

6. Transfer the skillet to the oven, and bake for 15 minutes, or until the potatoes are lightly browned.

SUBSTITUTION TIP: To make the recipe nut-free and allergen-free, use an unsweetened plain rice milk to make the potatoes and ensure that the dairy-free butter does not contain soy.

MEATLOAF

Make Gluten-Free, Nut-Free

SERVES 8

PREP TIME: 10 minutes COOK TIME: 1 hour, plus 10 minutes to rest

Some meatloaf recipes use milk-soaked bread crumbs or add Parmesan cheese. This version is just as delicious, but it uses diced tomatoes to keep the meatloaf moist. Tomatoes are lower in calories than dairy products, plus they add nice flavor, as do the fresh thyme and rosemary. I recommend baking the meatloaf directly on a sheet pan instead of the loaf pan, which helps it brown nicely all around.

1 tablespoon extra-virgin olive oil

1 yellow onion, minced

1 carrot, minced

1 celery stalk, minced

4 garlic cloves, minced

1 teaspoon minced fresh rosemary leaves

1 teaspoon minced fresh thyme leaves

Pinch red pepper flakes

½ cup toasted bread crumbs or gluten-free bread crumbs

1 egg

1 teaspoon sea salt

½ teaspoon freshly ground black pepper

2 plum tomatoes, finely diced (about ½ cup)

2 pounds ground beef

½ cup tomato ketchup, plus more for serving

Per Serving Calories: 310; Total Carbohydrates: 13g; Sugar: 6g; Total Fat: 20g; Saturated Fat: 7g; Sodium: 524mg; Protein: 22g; Fiber: 1g

1. Preheat the oven to 400°F. Line a rimmed sheet pan with parchment paper.

2. In a large skillet over medium heat, heat the oil. Add the onion, carrot, celery, garlic, rosemary, thyme, and red pepper flakes, and cook until soft, about 10 minutes. Allow to cool briefly.

3. In a large bowl, combine the bread crumbs, egg, salt, and pepper, and whisk to combine. Add the tomatoes and cooked vegetables, and stir until thoroughly mixed.

4. Add the ground beef, and use your hands to mix all the ingredients until just combined.

5. Spread the mixture into a 9-inch loaf pan to form, and then invert it onto the lined sheet pan. Drizzle with the ketchup and bake uncovered for 45 to 50 minutes or until the meatloaf is cooked through.

6. Allow the meatloaf to rest for 10 minutes, then slice into slightly larger than 1-inch-thick slices. Serve with additional ketchup.

INGREDIENT TIP: Onion, carrot, and celery are often used together in traditional French cooking and are referred to as mirepoix (meer-pwah).

BALSAMIC POT ROAST

Allergen-Free, Egg-Free, Gluten-Free, Nut-Free

SERVES 6

PREP TIME: 5 minutes
COOK TIME: 2 hours 45 minutes

This succulent pot roast gets basted with a tangy balsamic vinegar sauce. Although it takes a while to cook, most of the time is hands-off. You can also make it in a slow cooker (see Cooking tip). Serve with Scalloped Potatoes (page 83) and Sautéed Brussels Sprouts (page 77) for an elegant meal. This roast makes good leftovers, too—stuff it in toasted artisan rolls for a rich, flavorful sandwich.

2 tablespoons canola oil

1 (2-pound) boneless chuck roast

Sea salt

Freshly ground black pepper

1 red onion, halved and thinly sliced

1 rosemary sprig

1 cup balsamic vinegar

¼ cup brown sugar

2 cups beef broth

1 teaspoon Dijon mustard

Per Serving Calories: 507; Total Carbohydrates: 8g; Sugar: 7g; Total Fat: 39g; Saturated Fat: 14g; Sodium: 387mg; Protein: 29g; Fiber: 0g

1. Preheat the oven to 325°F.

2. In a large oven-safe skillet over medium-high heat, heat the oil.

3. Pat the roast dry with paper towels, and season generously with salt and pepper.

4. Sear the roast on all sides in the oil until well browned, 10 to 15 minutes.

5. Add the onion and rosemary to the pan.

6. In a small jar, whisk together the balsamic vinegar, sugar, broth, and mustard, and pour over the pot roast. Cover the skillet with a well-fitting lid and place in the oven.

7. Roast for 2 hours. Uncover, shred the meat with a fork, and return to the oven to cook uncovered for 30 more minutes.

COOKING TIP: To make this in a slow cooker, complete steps 1 through 4 and then place all the ingredients in the slow cooker. Cover and cook on high for 6 to 8 hours.

COFFEE-GLAZED STEAK

Allergen-Free, Egg-Free, Gluten-Free, Nut-Free

SERVES 4

PREP TIME: 5 minutes, plus 20 minutes to marinate COOK TIME: 40 minutes, plus 10 minutes to rest

This recipe is naturally dairy-free and came about on a girls' surf trip to Encinitas, California. We had a massive piece of steak in the refrigerator and a gas grill just waiting to cook it. The cupboards in the vacation rental were nearly bare, but I found some rum from the night before, leftover coffee, and a dusty spice rack. We also had a few odds and ends from making salad. Though invented in a pinch, the results far exceeded my expectations, and so here it is!

1½ cups strong brewed coffee, such as French press

½ cup dark rum

¼ cup red wine vinegar

¼ cup brown sugar

1 teaspoon coriander seeds

1 teaspoon peppercorns

1 large red onion, sliced

1 teaspoon sea salt

Freshly ground black pepper

1 (2-pound) hangar steak

1 teaspoon canola oil

Per Serving Calories: 427; Total Carbohydrates: 12g; Sugar: 10g; Total Fat: 10g; Saturated Fat: 0g; Sodium: 475mg; Protein: 52g; Fiber: 1g

1. In a medium saucepan over medium heat, combine the coffee, rum, vinegar, sugar, coriander, peppercorns, onion, salt, and a pinch pepper. Bring to a simmer and cook for 20 minutes, until reduced by about half. Allow the mixture to cool.

2. Pour half of the marinade over the steak, and allow to marinate for 20 minutes or up to 8 hours.

3. Preheat an outdoor grill to medium-high. Once hot, lightly coat the grates with oil using a folded paper towel.

4. Grill the steak for 5 to 10 minutes on each side, until cooked to your desired level of doneness. This will depend on the thickness of the steak and the grill's temperature.

5. Place the steak on a serving platter and drizzle with the remaining coffee glaze. Allow to rest for 10 minutes before slicing and serving.

SUBSTITUTION TIP: Feel free to use another tender cut of beef that does well with a short cooking time.

COOKING TIP: For convenience, step 1 can be done ahead of time.

STEAK AU POIVRE

Egg-Free, Gluten-Free, Make Allergen-Free, Nut-Free

SERVES 4

PREP TIME: 5 minutes   COOK TIME: 10 minutes

Coating steak in freshly ground pepper-corns and then pan searing is my favorite preparation method for steak because the pepper forms a nice crust on the browned meat. The traditional French recipe for peppercorn-crusted steak is called steak au poivre, or pepper steak, and is often served with a pan sauce made of heavy cream. This version uses a luxurious sauce created with cognac, dairy-free butter, and coconut cream.

4 (4- to 6-ounce) filet mignon steaks

¼ cup peppercorns, coarsely ground

½ teaspoon sea salt

1 tablespoon canola oil

¼ cup cognac or another brandy

2 tablespoons dairy-free butter, such as Earth Balance Buttery Spread

¼ cup store-bought coconut cream

Per Serving Calories: 483; Total Carbohydrates: 2g; Sugar: 1g; Total Fat: 29g; Saturated Fat: 11g; Sodium: 400mg; Protein: 49g; Fiber: 1g

1. Heat a large skillet over medium-high heat until very hot.

2. While the skillet heats, pat the steaks dry with paper towels, and season with the ground pepper and salt.

3. Add the oil to the hot skillet, and tilt to coat the bottom.

4. Sear the steaks in the skillet for 3 minutes on each side for medium-rare. Transfer the steaks to a cutting board to rest.

5. Carefully pour the cognac into the pan, and return it to the heat. Simmer for 2 minutes, until reduced to about 2 tablespoons.

6. Whisk in the dairy-free butter, and cook for 1 minute. Stir in the coconut cream, and simmer until just heated through and thick.

7. To serve, place the steaks on individual plates, and drizzle with the peppercorn pan sauce.

VARIATION TIP: Skip the brandy, dairy-free butter, and coconut cream, and opt for a lighter pan sauce that's also amazing with peppercorn-crusted steak. Add 1 cup of dry red wine and 2 thyme sprigs to the skillet after cooking the steak, and cook until reduced to about ⅓ cup, about 10 minutes.

BEEF STROGANOFF

Make Gluten-Free, Nut-Free

SERVES 5

PREP TIME: 10 minutes   COOK TIME: 25 minutes

I first enjoyed this flavorful beef stroganoff on Christmas Eve at my friend Christine's house. It was such a hit, I begged her for the recipe. There was something special about the meal that I couldn't put my finger on. It was bursting with flavor and all from a small addition of one "secret" ingredient: demi-glace. You can purchase it online or in well-stocked grocery stores, or make your own.

1 tablespoon canola oil

1 pound boneless rib-eye steak, thinly sliced on a bias

Sea salt

Freshly ground black pepper

1 yellow onion, halved and thinly sliced

1 tablespoon dairy-free butter, such as Earth Balance Buttery Spread

2 cups sliced cremini mushrooms

¼ cup brandy

1 cup beef broth

3 tablespoons demi-glace

1 bay leaf

1 teaspoon whole-grain mustard

½ cup Dairy-Free Sour Cream (page 192) or store-bought

12 ounces egg noodles or gluten-free noodles, cooked according to package directions

2 tablespoons roughly chopped fresh parsley

Per Serving Calories: 643; Total Carbohydrates: 54g; Sugar: 5g; Total Fat: 30g; Saturated Fat: 12g; Sodium: 358mg; Protein: 37g; Fiber: 3g

1. Heat a large skillet over medium-high heat. Add the oil, and tilt to coat the bottom.

2. Pat the rib-eye dry with paper towels, season it thoroughly with salt and pepper, and quickly sauté in the hot skillet until just cooked through, 3 to 5 minutes. Transfer the steak to a separate dish.

3. In the same pan, cook the onion until it begins to soften, about 5 minutes. Push it to the side, and add the dairy-free butter. When the dairy-free butter has melted, add the mushrooms, and allow to sear until well browned, about 10 minutes.

4. Carefully pour in the brandy and deglaze the pan, scraping up the browned bits.

5. Return the steak, along with any accumulated juices, to the skillet. Add the broth, demi-glace, bay leaf, and mustard, and simmer for 5 minutes.

continued ☞

6. Remove the skillet from the heat, remove and discard the bay leaf, and stir in the dairy-free sour cream until integrated into the sauce. Stir in the cooked egg noodles.

7. Sprinkle with the parsley to serve.

SUBSTITUTION TIP: Egg noodles are a common addition to beef stroganoff in the United States, but mashed potatoes are a more traditional accompaniment in Russia. For an egg-free and naturally gluten-free starch, make mashed potatoes with potato flakes, unsweetened almond milk, and dairy-free butter.

MONGOLIAN BEEF

Egg-Free, Make Allergen-Free, Make Gluten-Free, Nut-Free

SERVES 4

PREP TIME: 5 minutes   COOK TIME: 5 minutes

This tangy, spicy dish is naturally dairy-free and so easy to whip up at home, making it an excellent addition to your weeknight menu rotation. When you make it yourself, you can choose your ingredients, making it much healthier than restaurant versions. This version dramatically reduces the sugar content and oil, and if you'd like to make it gluten-free, use gluten-free soy sauce.

1 pound flank steak, thinly sliced on a bias

Sea salt

Freshly ground black pepper

2 tablespoons cornstarch

2 tablespoons canola oil

1 tablespoon minced fresh ginger

1 tablespoon minced garlic

⅛ teaspoon red pepper flakes

½ cup low-sodium soy sauce

2 tablespoons hoisin sauce

2 tablespoons brown sugar

4 scallions, cut in 2-inch pieces

Steamed white rice, for serving

Per Serving Calories: 378; Total Carbohydrates: 16g; Sugar: 9g; Total Fat: 20g; Saturated Fat: 6g; Sodium: 2047mg; Protein: 34g; Fiber: 1g

1. Season the flank steak with salt and pepper, and put in a bowl. Add the cornstarch, and toss gently to coat the meat.

2. Heat a large wok or skillet over high heat. When hot, add the oil.

3. Sear the beef until browned and just cooked through, 3 to 4 minutes. Transfer to a separate dish.

4. Reduce the heat to medium-low, and add the ginger, garlic, and red pepper flakes to the wok. Cook until fragrant, about 30 seconds.

5. Add the soy sauce, hoisin sauce, and sugar, and stir until the sugar is dissolved.

6. Add the scallions and beef, and simmer for 1 more minute, just until the scallions are wilted. Serve with white rice.

INGREDIENT TIP: You can find hoisin sauce in the Asian section of most grocery stores or purchase it online.

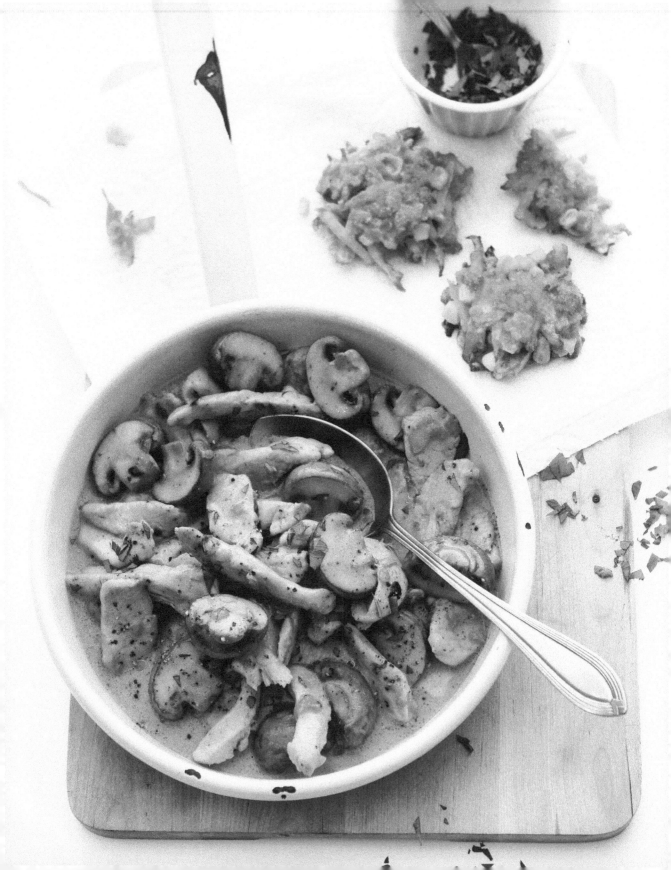

POULTRY

Pan-Seared Chicken with Mushrooms and Cream, page 132

HERB AND GARLIC ROASTED CHICKEN

Allergen-Free, Egg-Free, Gluten-Free, Nut-Free

SERVES 5

PREP TIME: 5 minutes   COOK TIME: 45 minutes, plus 10 minutes to rest

Winner, winner, chicken dinner. This recipe has it all—it's easy and flavorful, and it feeds a lot of hungry mouths. Most nights, it also yields leftovers. Have your butcher spatchcock the chicken for you, or do it yourself (see the Cooking tip).

1 (3- to 4-pound) whole chicken, spatchcocked

2 tablespoons extra-virgin olive oil

1 tablespoon minced garlic

¼ cup minced fresh herbs, such as parsley, rosemary, and thyme

½ teaspoon finely grated lemon zest

Sea salt

Freshly ground black pepper

Per Serving Calories: 628; Total Carbohydrates: 0g; Sugar: 0g; Total Fat: 49g; Saturated Fat: 13g; Sodium: 229mg; Protein: 46g; Fiber: 0g

1. Preheat the oven to 400°F.

2. Place the chicken cut-side down on a large sheet pan. Flatten it with your hands by pressing down between the breasts.

3. In a small jar, whisk together the oil, garlic, herbs, and lemon zest. Pour the mixture over the chicken, rubbing it over both sides and pressing the mixture up under the skin. Season with salt and pepper.

4. Roast the chicken for 45 minutes or until it reaches an internal temperature of 160°F. It will continue cooking after it is removed from the oven.

5. Allow the chicken to rest for 10 minutes before carving and serving.

COOKING TIP: To remove the backbone from the chicken, balance it on one end, with the breasts facing away from you, in the kitchen sink. Using a sharp serrated knife or kitchen shears, cut down one side of the backbone, then cut down the other side. Remove the backbone and use it for making stock.

CHICKEN IN WHITE WINE

Egg-Free, Gluten-Free, Make Allergen-Free, Nut-Free

SERVES 4

PREP TIME: 5 minutes COOK TIME: 30 minutes

This classic French recipe for coq au vin can be made with red or white wine, but I prefer the subtlety of white wine. Plus, it doesn't stain the chicken purple. The sauce is typically finished with butter, but in this version, I reduce it further on the stove top and whisk in a dairy-free butter to yield a rich, velvety sauce.

1 tablespoon canola oil

1 pound boneless, skinless chicken thighs

Sea salt

Freshly ground black pepper

1 cup minced yellow onion

2 garlic cloves, smashed

1 thyme sprig

1½ cups dry white wine

1 cup low-sodium chicken broth

2 tablespoons dairy-free butter, such as Earth Balance Buttery Spread

Per Serving Calories: 302; Total Carbohydrates: 6g; Sugar: 2g; Total Fat: 14g; Saturated Fat: 3g; Sodium: 237mg; Protein: 23g; Fiber: 1g

1. Place a large pot over medium-high heat. When it is hot, add the oil.

2. Pat the chicken thighs dry with paper towels, and season generously with salt and pepper.

3. Sear the chicken in the hot oil until just browned on each side but not cooked through, about 2 minutes per side. Remove to a separate dish.

4. Add the onion and garlic to the pot, and cook for 3 minutes, until just beginning to soften. Add the thyme.

5. Return the chicken and any accumulated juices to the pot. Add the wine and broth. Bring to a gentle simmer and cook for 15 minutes, or until the chicken is cooked through.

6. Transfer the chicken to a serving platter, and simmer the remaining pot liquid until it has reduced to about 1 cup, about 8 minutes. Remove and discard the thyme, and whisk in the dairy-free butter. Pour the sauce over the chicken.

COOKING TIP: Some recipes for coq au vin call for using skin-on chicken pieces, but I found that even after a perfect sear, the skin becomes slimy after being cooked in wine. Not too appetizing!

BARBECUE CHICKEN RANCH PIZZA

Egg-Free, Make Gluten-Free, Nut-Free

SERVES 2

PREP TIME: 10 minutes COOK TIME: 10 to 12 minutes

It sounds like junk food heaven, but this pizza is actually pretty healthy. Grilled chicken, a low-sugar barbecue sauce, and dairy-free ranch dressing atop a whole-grain crust make for a surprisingly sensible but yummy dinner. I suggest adding some thinly sliced spinach and scallions for color and texture, if you're so inclined.

1 (12-inch) prepared whole-grain or gluten-free pizza crust

1 cup low-sugar barbecue sauce, such as Stubb's (see Ingredient tip)

8 ounces grilled chicken, sliced

½ red onion, thinly sliced

½ cup Ranch Dressing (page 188)

½ cup thinly sliced spinach (optional)

1 scallion, thinly sliced on a bias (optional)

Per Serving Calories: 443; Total Carbohydrates: 44g; Sugar: 21g; Total Fat: 4g; Saturated Fat: 1g; Sodium: 1670mg; Protein: 58g; Fiber: 2g

1. Preheat the oven to 400°F.

2. Place the pizza crust on a large sheet pan, and spread the top with the barbecue sauce. Layer the chicken and onion over the sauce.

3. Bake for 10 to 12 minutes, until the sauce is hot and bubbling and the crust begins to brown. Remove the pizza from the oven.

4. Drizzle with the ranch dressing, and sprinkle with the spinach (if using) and scallions (if using) before serving.

INGREDIENT TIP: When I'm not making it from scratch, my favorite brand of barbecue sauce is Stubb's. It is naturally gluten-free and has only 2 to 4 grams of sugar per serving depending on which variety you choose, which is a fraction of the sugar in other brands.

GREEN CHILE CHICKEN ENCHILADAS

Allergen-Free, Egg-Free, Gluten-Free, Nut-Free

SERVES 4

PREP TIME: 10 minutes COOK TIME: 30 minutes, plus 5 minutes to rest

The timeless Mexican dish has endured the ages, and if you're worried that it can't be as good as the cheesy version, rest assured that these are fabulous. In fact, cheese was only introduced to enchiladas after many generations of enchiladas focused on meat, tomatoes, and chiles. In this recipe, tangy green sauce envelops these enchiladas stuffed with chicken, peppers, onions, garlic, and dairy-free cream cheese.

1 tablespoon canola oil, plus more for coating the casserole

1 pound boneless, skinless chicken thighs, diced

Sea salt

Freshly ground black pepper

1 green bell pepper, cored and thinly sliced

1 small yellow onion, halved and thinly sliced

1 tablespoon minced garlic

1 (8-ounce) container dairy-free cream cheese

12 corn tortillas

1 (15-ounce) can green chile enchilada sauce

Per Serving Calories: 423; Total Carbohydrates: 20g; Sugar: 6g; Total Fat: 31g; Saturated Fat: 10g; Sodium: 1304mg; Protein: 19g; Fiber: 1g

1. Preheat the oven to 375°F. Lightly coat a 2-quart casserole dish with oil.

2. In a large skillet over medium-high heat, heat the remaining 1 tablespoon of oil. Season the chicken with salt and pepper. Add the chicken to the skillet and cook for 2 minutes, stirring occasionally.

3. Add the bell pepper and onion to the skillet, and cook, stirring occasionally, for another 7 to 8 minutes, until the vegetables are soft and the chicken is cooked through. Add the garlic and cook for another 30 seconds, until fragrant.

4. Stir in the dairy-free cream cheese, giving everything a good toss to mix.

5. Heat the corn tortillas individually in the microwave for about 10 seconds each, or until they're pliable. Scoop a heaping ¼ cup of warm filling into a tortilla and roll into a cylinder. Place it in the casserole dish. Repeat with the remaining filling and tortillas.

6. Pour the enchilada sauce over the enchiladas, and bake for 20 minutes. Allow to rest for 5 minutes before serving.

COOKING TIP: You can prepare this dish ahead of time and refrigerate until ready to bake. Add 10 minutes to the cooking time.

PAN-SEARED CHICKEN WITH MUSHROOMS AND CREAM

Allergen-Free, Egg-Free, Gluten-Free, Nut-Free

SERVES 4

PREP TIME: 5 minutes COOK TIME: 15 minutes

Decadent, creamy, and filled with umami flavors, this chicken dish is far greater than the sum of its parts. The recipe, inspired by the classic French recipe for mushrooms in port and cream, takes a fraction of the time, and swaps butter and cream for canola oil and coconut cream for a comparable dairy-free option. Serve with Sautéed Brussels Sprouts (page 77) or Rosemary Roasted Potatoes (page 82).

2 tablespoons canola oil, divided

4 (4-ounce) boneless, skinless chicken thighs

Sea salt

Freshly ground black pepper

2 cups thinly sliced cremini mushrooms

1 small shallot, minced

¼ cup port

¼ cup store-bought coconut cream

Per Serving Calories: 321; Total Carbohydrates: 5g; Sugar: 1g; Total Fat: 22g; Saturated Fat: 10g; Sodium: 161mg; Protein: 24g; Fiber: 0g

1. Heat a large skillet over medium-high heat. Add 1 tablespoon of oil, and tilt to coat the bottom.

2. Season the chicken on all sides with salt and pepper. Sear the chicken in the skillet on each side for 2 minutes, until browned but not cooked through. Transfer to a separate dish.

3. Add the remaining 1 tablespoon of oil to the skillet, and cook the mushrooms and shallot for 5 minutes, until the mushrooms are deeply browned.

4. Add the port, cooking for 1 minute to burn off some of the alcohol. Add the coconut cream, and bring to a simmer.

5. Return the chicken and any accumulated juices to the skillet, and cook until the chicken is cooked through and the sauce is thick, about 2 more minutes.

COOKING TIP: Want even more mushroomy goodness? Soak 1 ounce of dried wild mushrooms in 1 cup of boiling water for 10 minutes. Strain the mushrooms, reserving the broth for another use. Roughly chop the mushrooms, and add them during the last minute of the fresh mushroom cooking time.

CREAMY COCONUT-LIME CHICKEN

Allergen-Free, Egg-Free, Gluten-Free, Nut-Free

SERVES 4

PREP TIME: 10 minutes COOK TIME: 20 minutes

This one-pan supper hits all the right notes. It's tangy, spicy, and creamy, with just a hint of sweetness. The flavor of the coconut milk is a welcome addition, so I don't recommend swapping it for another non-dairy milk.

1 tablespoon canola oil

4 (6-ounce) boneless, skinless chicken breasts

Sea salt

Freshly ground black pepper

½ red onion, halved and thinly sliced

2 garlic cloves, smashed

1 teaspoon minced ginger

Pinch red pepper flakes

1 cup coconut milk

½ cup chicken broth

12 ounces green beans, trimmed

Zest and juice of 1 lime

¼ cup roughly chopped fresh cilantro

Per Serving Calories: 390; Total Carbohydrates: 12g; Sugar: 4g; Total Fat: 20g; Saturated Fat: 13g; Sodium: 282mg; Protein: 43g; Fiber: 5g

1. In a large skillet over medium-high heat, heat the oil.

2. Pat the chicken dry with paper towels and season with salt and pepper. Sear the chicken in the skillet for 4 to 5 minutes on one side, until well browned. Flip the chicken.

3. Add the onion, garlic, ginger, and red pepper flakes to the pan. Cook for 2 minutes, until fragrant.

4. Add the coconut milk, broth, green beans, and lime zest (reserve the lime juice). Simmer for 10 minutes, until the chicken is cooked through and the green beans are tender.

5. Stir in the lime juice and cilantro, and serve.

INGREDIENT TIP: For the best texture, purchase young, thin green beans such as haricots verts for this recipe.

CREAMY GREEN GODDESS CHICKEN

Egg-Free, Gluten-Free

SERVES 4

PREP TIME: 5 minutes COOK TIME: 10 minutes

Originating in San Francisco in the 1920s, Green Goddess dressing was created by chef Philip Roemer of the Palace Hotel as a tribute to a play by the same name. The sauce is remarkably similar to the French sauce *au vert*, which also contains tarragon, lemon juice, and parsley. Whatever its origins, the bright, springtime flavors in this dish are perfectly balanced by the creaminess of the cashew cream. You can also use another unsweetened dairy-free creamer.

1 tablespoon canola oil

4 (6-ounce) boneless, skinless chicken breasts

Sea salt

Freshly ground black pepper

1 small shallot, minced

¼ cup fresh parsley leaves and tender stems

2 tablespoons minced fresh chives

2 tablespoons minced fresh tarragon

1 teaspoon freshly squeezed lemon juice

¼ cup Cashew Cream (page 22)

¼ cup chicken broth

Per Serving Calories: 253; Total Carbohydrates: 2g; Sugar: 1g; Total Fat: 10g; Saturated Fat: 4g; Sodium: 222mg; Protein: 40g; Fiber: 1g

1. Heat a large skillet over medium-high heat. Add the oil, and tilt to coat the bottom.

2. Season the chicken on all sides with salt and pepper. Sear the chicken in the skillet on one side for 5 minutes, until well browned.

3. While the chicken cooks, in a blender, combine the shallot, parsley, chives, tarragon, lemon juice, cashew cream, and chicken broth. Purée until smooth.

4. Flip the chicken and sear for 5 minutes on the other side, until cooked through.

5. Add the dressing to the pan with the chicken, and cook until just warmed.

COOKING TIP: Delicate fresh herbs such as tarragon lose their flavor when cooked for prolonged periods. Adding the sauce at the end warms it gently while preserving the flavor.

CREAMY SUN-DRIED TOMATO CHICKEN FETTUCINE

Allergen-Free, Egg-Free, Make Gluten-Free, Nut-Free

SERVES 4

PREP TIME: 5 minutes COOK TIME: 15 minutes

Sun-dried tomatoes enliven this creamy chicken dish made with sautéed red onions, garlic, and fresh oregano. The creamy texture of the coconut cream works nicely in this dish, but its tropical undertones are completely upstaged by the pungent flavor of garlic and herbs. This dish is especially awesome served over the bed of fresh pasta.

12 ounces fettucine noodles or gluten-free pasta

1 tablespoon canola oil

1 pound boneless, skinless chicken pieces

Sea salt

Freshly ground black pepper

½ red onion, thinly sliced

2 garlic cloves, smashed

½ cup thinly sliced, oil-packed sun-dried tomatoes, drained

2 teaspoons minced fresh oregano

1 cup chicken broth

¼ cup store-bought coconut cream

1 cup thinly sliced fresh spinach

¼ cup roughly chopped fresh basil

Per Serving Calories: 563; Total Carbohydrates: 71g; Sugar: 4g; Total Fat: 14g; Saturated Fat: 4g; Sodium: 358mg; Protein: 38g; Fiber: 5g

1. Bring a large pot of salted water to a boil. Cook the pasta according to the package instructions, about 10 minutes.

2. While it is cooking, heat a large skillet over medium-high heat. Add the oil, and tilt to coat the bottom.

3. Season the chicken on all sides with salt and pepper. Sear the chicken in the skillet for 2 minutes on one side.

4. Flip the chicken pieces, and add the onion, garlic, tomatoes, oregano, and broth. Bring to a simmer and cook for 10 minutes, until the chicken is cooked through.

5. Add the coconut cream to the pan, and cook for another minute.

6. Just before serving, stir in the fresh spinach and basil. Place the pasta in a serving dish and pour the chicken and sauce over the top.

SUBSTITUTION TIP: To reduce the fat in this dish, use dry-packed sun-dried tomatoes.

CITRUS BACON CHICKEN

Egg-Free, Gluten-Free, Nut-Free

SERVES 4

PREP TIME: 5 minutes COOK TIME: 25 minutes

Citrus and bacon sound like an odd pairing, but they are so good together! Think breakfast bacon and orange juice, but better. The bacon renders its smoky fat into the pan for cooking the chicken and then the freshly squeezed orange juice reduces to a syrupy glaze for a perfect balance of salty, sour, and sweet.

2 applewood smoked bacon slices, roughly chopped

4 boneless, skinless chicken breasts, pounded to a uniform ½-inch thickness

Sea salt

Freshly ground black pepper

1 cup freshly squeezed orange juice

1 tablespoon freshly squeezed lime juice

2 tablespoons honey

2 scallions, green parts only, very thinly sliced on a bias

Per Serving Calories: 244; Total Carbohydrates: 17g; Sugar: 14g; Total Fat: 7g; Saturated Fat: 1g; Sodium: 337mg; Protein: 28g; Fiber: 0g

1. Heat a large skillet over medium-low heat. Cook the bacon until it renders most of its fat, about 10 minutes. Transfer the bacon to a dish, leaving the fat in the pan.

2. Increase the heat to medium-high. Pat the chicken breasts dry with paper towels and season generously with salt and pepper. Sear the chicken in the skillet on each side for 4 minutes, or until just cooked through. Transfer to a separate dish (not with the bacon).

3. Add the orange juice, lime juice, and honey to the skillet, and simmer until reduced to about ½ cup of liquid, about 5 minutes.

4. Return the chicken to the skillet and turn to coat in the sauce. Remove from the heat.

5. Place each chicken breast on a serving plate, and top with a couple tablespoons of the sauce. Sprinkle with the cooked bacon and scallions.

   INGREDIENT TIP: If you can find them, add ½ cup of thinly sliced kumquats to the skillet when you add the orange juice. They have a bracing acidity that mellows slightly as they cook and adds complexity to the sauce.

BACON-WRAPPED CHICKEN

Allergen-Free, Egg-Free, Gluten-Free, Nut-Free

SERVES 4

PREP TIME: 5 minutes   COOK TIME: 30 minutes

Four ingredients and just five minutes of prep time make this chicken dinner a perfect weeknight supper. It also lends itself well to prepping ahead of time and simply placing in the oven when you're ready to eat. Serve this dish with Polenta Fries (page 73), which can be baked on the same pan.

4 (6-ounce) boneless, skinless chicken breasts

Sea salt

Freshly ground black pepper

1 tablespoon minced fresh rosemary leaves

1 tablespoon minced garlic

8 applewood smoked bacon slices

Per Serving Calories: 391; Total Carbohydrates: 2g; Sugar: 0g; Total Fat: 18g; Saturated Fat: 5g; Sodium: 1050mg; Protein: 53g; Fiber: 0g

1. Preheat the oven to 400°F. Line a sheet pan with parchment paper.

2. Season each chicken breast liberally with salt and pepper, then coat with the rosemary and garlic.

3. Wrap each chicken breast in 2 slices of bacon, and place them seam-side down on the pan.

4. Bake for 30 minutes, or until the chicken is cooked through and the bacon has rendered most of its fat.

SUBSTITUTION TIP: This recipe works best with fresh herbs. If you're not a fan of rosemary, try basil, tarragon, or thyme.

CASHEW, CHICKEN, AND MANGO STIR-FRY

Egg-Free, Gluten-Free

SERVES 4

PREP TIME: 5 minutes COOK TIME: 10 to 15 minutes

I have been making some rendition of this dish for years. There's something about the spicy red pepper flakes, sweet mango, salty fish sauce, and crunchy snap peas that just works for me. It's naturally low in carbs, but you can serve it with steamed rice for a complete meal.

1 tablespoon canola oil

1 pound boneless, skinless chicken thighs, diced

2 tablespoons fish sauce

2 tablespoons freshly squeezed lime juice

1 tablespoon brown sugar

1 pound sugar snap peas, stringed and halved

2 garlic cloves, minced

⅛ teaspoon red pepper flakes

½ cup toasted cashews

1 mango, diced

Per Serving Calories: 484; Total Carbohydrates: 31g; Sugar: 20g; Total Fat: 29g; Saturated Fat: 7g; Sodium: 789mg; Protein: 27g; Fiber: 5g

1. In a large skillet over medium-high heat, heat the oil, and tilt to coat the bottom.

2. Add the chicken thighs and cook, stirring occasionally, for 6 to 8 minutes, until just cooked through. Transfer to a separate dish.

3. While the chicken cooks, in a small bowl, whisk together the fish sauce, lime juice, and sugar. Set aside.

4. Add the snap peas to the skillet, and cook for 2 to 3 minutes, until bright green.

5. Add the garlic and red pepper flakes, and cook until fragrant, about 30 seconds.

6. Pour the fish sauce mixture back into the skillet, and return the chicken and any accumulated juices to the skillet also.

7. Cook for 30 seconds and then remove from the heat. Carefully fold in the cashews and mango. Serve immediately.

COOKING TIP: It's best to have all of the ingredients measured ahead of time, because this dish comes together really quickly!

CHICKEN TIKKA MASALA

Allergen-Free, Egg-Free, Gluten-Free, Nut-Free

PREP TIME: 10 minutes COOK TIME: 15 minutes

When I lived in England, tikka masala was my favorite thing to eat when we went out to the pub. I could find it right alongside bangers and mash and fish and chips, but it was far more flavorful and healthier, too. Not the history you envisioned from the name, right? Its origin is debated, but it remains a British favorite. Traditionally, the dish is thickened with yogurt and heavy cream, but this version uses coconut cream, which pairs well with the fragrant Indian spices.

1 tablespoon canola oil

1 yellow onion, diced

2 garlic cloves, minced

1 teaspoon minced fresh ginger

1 teaspoon ground coriander

1 teaspoon ground cumin

1 teaspoon smoked paprika

⅛ teaspoon red pepper flakes

1 pound boneless, skinless chicken thighs

1 (15-ounce) can diced plum tomatoes

1 cup low-sodium chicken broth

Sea salt

Freshly ground black pepper

¼ cup store-bought coconut cream

¼ cup minced fresh cilantro

1 lime, cut into wedges, for serving

Per Serving Calories: 347; Total Carbohydrates: 9g; Sugar: 5g; Total Fat: 25g; Saturated Fat: 9g; Sodium: 171mg; Protein: 22g; Fiber: 3g

1. In a large skillet over medium heat, heat the oil.

2. Cook the onion, garlic, and ginger for 5 minutes, until the onion has somewhat softened.

3. Add the coriander, cumin, paprika, and red pepper flakes to the skillet, and cook for 1 minute, until fragrant.

4. Add the chicken to the skillet, along with the tomatoes and broth. Season generously with salt and pepper. Simmer until the chicken is cooked through, about 10 minutes.

5. Remove the skillet from the heat, and stir in the coconut cream. Garnish with the cilantro and serve with lime wedges.

COOKING TIP: This recipe also works in a slow cooker. Combine all the ingredients except the coconut cream and cilantro, and cook on low for 6 to 8 hours. Stir in the coconut cream and cilantro just before serving.

SOUTHWESTERN CHICKEN CASSEROLE

Allergen-Free, Egg-Free, Gluten-Free, Nut-Free

SERVES 4

PREP TIME: 5 minutes   COOK TIME: 35 minutes

This easy, one-dish main dish is inspired by a stuffed chicken breast I enjoyed at a modern Mexican restaurant in Arizona. Stuffing individual chicken breasts can be time-consuming and a little fussy for my taste. Plus, the chicken easily dries out before the filling has a chance to cook. So instead, I turned it into this creamy casserole. Serve this with blue corn tortilla chips.

1 teaspoon canola oil

2 cups shredded cooked chicken breast

2 cups cooked white or brown rice

1 cup fresh corn kernels

¼ cup diced green chiles

¼ cup minced sun-dried tomatoes

1 cup Dairy-Free Sour Cream (page 192) or store-bought

¼ cup minced fresh cilantro

Sea salt

Freshly ground black pepper

Per Serving Calories: 404; Total Carbohydrates: 41g; Sugar: 7g; Total Fat: 15g; Saturated Fat: 11g; Sodium: 298mg; Protein: 26g; Fiber: 2g

1. Preheat the oven to 400°F. Coat the interior of a 2-quart casserole dish with the oil.

2. Add the chicken, rice, corn, chiles, tomatoes, and sour cream to the dish, and toss gently to mix. Flatten with the back of a spatula.

3. Bake uncovered for 35 minutes, until the casserole is golden brown and bubbling. Top with the cilantro to serve, and season with salt and pepper.

INGREDIENT TIP: I like to purchase a whole rotisserie chicken to use in this recipe. I have plenty left over for other meals and can use the bones to make stock.

CHICKEN CASSOULET

Allergen-Free, Egg-Free, Gluten-Free, Nut-Free

SERVES 5

PREP TIME: 10 minutes   COOK TIME: 55 minutes

Cassoulet is a rich, warming French stew of pork, chicken or duck, sausage, and white beans. The traditional method is precise and involved—think six hours of active cooking time! However, with a few shortcuts you can recreate the succulent flavors and exquisite texture of classic cassoulet in a fraction of the time.

4 ounces salt pork, cut into lardons (strips) or cubes

1 pound bone-in chicken thighs

1 pound chicken drumsticks

Sea salt

Freshly ground black pepper

2 garlic sausage links, casings removed, crumbled

1 small yellow onion, minced

2 carrots, minced

2 celery stalks, minced

6 garlic cloves, smashed

2 (15-ounce) cans cannellini beans, drained

2 bay leaves

4 cups chicken broth

¼ cup dry white wine

Per Serving Calories: 726; Total Carbohydrates: 38g; Sugar: 6g; Total Fat: 40g; Saturated Fat: 12g; Sodium: 2181mg; Protein: 50g; Fiber: 12g

1. Preheat the oven to 425°F.

2. Heat a large cast iron skillet or Dutch oven over medium heat. Cook the pork until it renders most of its fat, about 10 minutes. Transfer the pork to a dish, leaving the fat in the pan.

3. Increase the heat to high. Pat the chicken thighs and drumsticks dry with paper towels and season with salt and pepper. Sear in the skillet for 3 minutes on each side, until gently browned. Transfer the chicken to a separate dish (not with the pork).

4. Add the sausage to the skillet, and cook for 4 minutes. Push the sausage to the side and add the onion, carrots, celery, and garlic to the skillet. Cook for 5 minutes.

5. Add the pork, beans, bay leaves, broth, and wine, and bring to a simmer.

6. Place the chicken pieces skin-side up on top of the beans, and transfer the skillet to the oven. Bake for 30 minutes, until the meat is deeply browned.

INGREDIENT TIP: Read the label to make sure the garlic sausages do not contain dairy.

SERVING TIP: Take the night off from cleanup—whoever finds a bay leaf has to do the dishes.

CUBAN CHICKEN STEW

Allergen-Free, Egg-Free, Gluten-Free, Nut-Free

SERVES 4

PREP TIME: 10 minutes COOK TIME: 35 minutes

The flavors in this sweet and tangy stew might seem to be a strange combination, but they totally work. It's a one-pot meal that easily doubles to feed a crowd. Sop the juices up with some *pan Cubano* (Cuban bread) or a loaf of French bread for a complete meal.

2 tablespoons extra-virgin olive oil

1 onion, halved and thinly sliced

1 green bell pepper, cored and thinly sliced

4 garlic cloves, smashed

1 pound boneless, skinless chicken thighs

Sea salt

Freshly ground black pepper

½ cup dry white wine

1 teaspoon ground cumin

1 teaspoon dried oregano

2 cups peeled and diced potatoes

2 tablespoons tomato paste

2 cups chicken broth

Zest and juice of 1 lime

Zest and juice of 1 orange

1 cup frozen peas, thawed

¼ cup raisins

¼ cup halved, pitted green olives

2 tablespoons drained capers

2 tablespoons chopped fresh parsley

Per Serving Calories: 583; Total Carbohydrates: 41g; Sugar: 12g; Total Fat: 31g; Saturated Fat: 8g; Sodium: 1633mg; Protein: 29g; Fiber: 7g

1. In a large skillet over medium-high heat, heat the oil.

2. Add the onion, bell pepper, and garlic to the skillet, and cook for 5 minutes.

3. Pat the chicken thighs dry with paper towels, and season generously with salt and pepper.

4. Push the vegetables to the side of the skillet and add the chicken. Cook for 5 minutes, until just beginning to brown.

5. Add the wine and deglaze the pan, scraping up the browned bits.

6. Stir in the cumin, oregano, potatoes, tomato paste, broth, lime zest and juice, and orange zest and juice. Bring to a simmer, cover, and cook for 20 minutes, until the potatoes are tender.

7. Uncover, and stir in the peas, raisins, olives, and capers. Cook for another 5 minutes.

8. Garnish with the parsley and serve.

   COOKING TIP: This dish also works well in a slow cooker. Place all the ingredients in the slow cooker and cook on low for 8 hours.

TURKEY MUSHROOM STEW

Egg-Free, Gluten-Free

SERVES 4

PREP TIME: 5 minutes COOK TIME: 15 minutes

My favorite season for cooking is fall, when the leaves turn golden brown, the days become shorter, and the air has a brisk chill. Here in California, this glorious transition begins in September, although sweater season doesn't come for weeks afterward. But that doesn't stop me from breaking out all of my favorite stew recipes the moment Labor Day passes. This creamy turkey mushroom stew is one of my favorites. Serve with Sweet Potato Corn Cakes (page 78) and a dark beer.

2 tablespoons dairy-free butter, such as Earth Balance Buttery Spread

2 cups halved cremini mushrooms

1 small shallot, minced

1 teaspoon minced fresh thyme leaves

1 pound boneless, skinless turkey cutlets

Sea salt

Freshly ground black pepper

2 tablespoons all-purpose flour or gluten-free flour blend

1 tablespoon canola oil

2 tablespoons dry sherry

½ cup Cashew Cream (page 22)

1 cup chicken broth

¼ cup minced fresh parsley

Per Serving Calories: 329; Total Carbohydrates: 7g; Sugar: 1g; Total Fat: 18g; Saturated Fat: 9g; Sodium: 382mg; Protein: 30g; Fiber: 1g

1. In a large, deep skillet over medium-high heat, heat the dairy-free butter.

2. Add the mushrooms and cook for 5 minutes, until well browned. Add the shallot and thyme, and cook for another minute. Push the vegetables to the side of the skillet.

3. Season the turkey with salt and pepper. Pour the flour into a wide, shallow bowl and turn the turkey in the flour to coat.

4. Add the oil to the skillet. Add the turkey and cook for 5 minutes, until just cooked through.

5. Pour in the sherry and cook for 30 seconds, scraping up the browned bits from the bottom of the pan.

6. Add the cashew cream and broth, and bring to a simmer. Cook for 2 to 3 minutes, until just thickened. Top with the parsley and a few grinds of black pepper.

INGREDIENT TIP: Cremini mushrooms, also called baby bellas, can be replaced with button mushrooms if needed, but their earthy flavor is worth seeking out at your local supermarket.

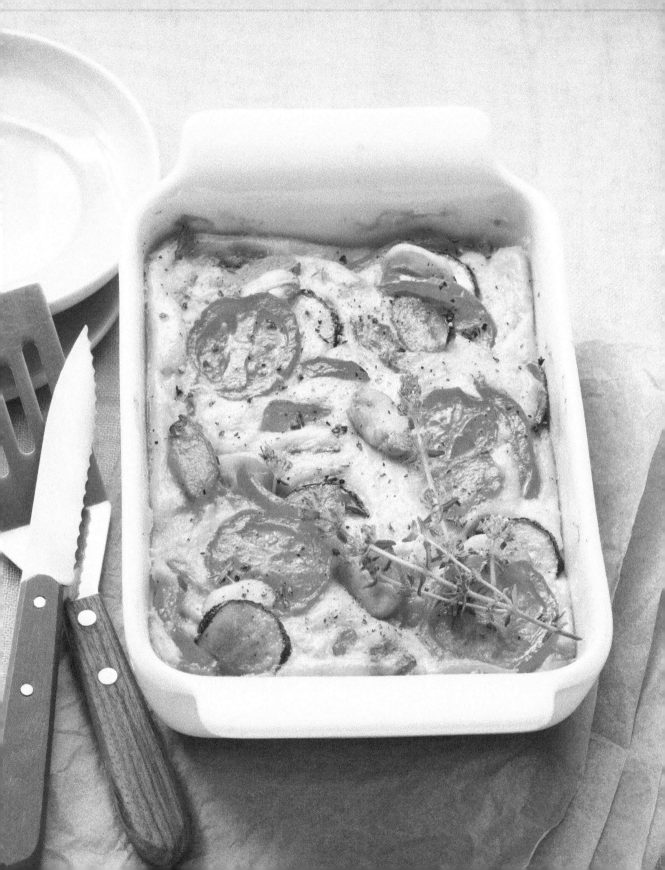

Chapter Ten

VEGETARIAN AND VEGAN

Creamy Polenta Vegetable Bake, page 156

DEEP DISH VEGGIE PIZZA

Egg-Free, Make Gluten-Free, Nut-Free, Vegan

SERVES 2 TO 4

PREP TIME: 10 minutes COOK TIME: 25 minutes, plus 10 minutes to rest

Late one Sunday afternoon, Brad asked for pizza for dinner. I didn't think I had any of the ingredients in the kitchen—just fresh tomatoes from the school garden, an assortment of gluten-free flours, and a block of tofu. What followed has to be one of my greatest mom triumphs in the kitchen. I whipped together a gluten-free pizza dough, made an epic pomodoro sauce, and topped it all with fresh tofu ricotta and plenty of fresh basil, olives, onions, and peppers. I thought the pizza alone was enough cause to celebrate, but when Brad said, "This is vegan? It is mind-blowing!" I was thrilled.

1 tablespoon extra-virgin olive oil

1 tablespoon ground cornmeal

1 pizza dough (suitable for a 12-inch pizza)

1 cup Pomodoro Sauce (page 195) or good-quality store-bought marinara sauce

1 cup Tofu Ricotta (page 29)

½ cup thinly sliced green bell peppers

½ cup thinly sliced red onion

¼ cup roughly chopped, pitted Kalamata olives

¼ cup minced fresh basil

2 tablespoons Plant-Based Parmesan (page 27, optional)

Per Serving Calories: 206; Total Carbohydrates: 23g; Sugar: 8g; Total Fat: 10g; Saturated Fat: 3g; Sodium: 520mg; Protein: 8g; Fiber: 3g

1. Preheat the oven to 425°F.

2. Coat the interior of a cast iron skillet with the oil and sprinkle with the cornmeal.

3. Stretch the pizza dough and place it in the skillet, pressing any excess dough up the sides of the skillet.

4. Par-bake the crust according to the package instructions, about 10 minutes.

5. Spread the sauce over the crust and top with dollops of tofu ricotta. Sprinkle the bell peppers, onion, and olives over the pizza.

6. Bake for 15 minutes, or until the ricotta is lightly browned. Allow the pizza to rest for 10 minutes before topping with the basil and plant-based Parmesan (if using). Slice and serve.

COOKING TIP: For an excellent gluten-free pizza dough, check out my book *The Gluten-Free Cookbook for Families*, which includes a recipe for a quick-rising pizza dough made with almond flour.

CREAMY ARTICHOKE AND PESTO PIZZA

Egg-Free, Make Gluten-Free, Make Nut-Free, Vegan

SERVES 2 TO 5

PREP TIME: 10 minutes COOK TIME: 20 minutes, plus 10 minutes to rest

I really can't decide which I like better—the traditional Deep Dish Veggie Pizza (page 146) with its classic pomodoro sauce or this flavorful pesto pizza topped with creamy cheese sauce and marinated artichoke hearts. But why choose? They're both awesome.

2 tablespoons extra-virgin olive oil, divided

1 tablespoon cornmeal

1 pizza dough (suitable for a 12-inch pizza)

1 leek, halved and thinly sliced

Pinch sea salt

1 cup Spinach-Basil Pesto (page 193)

1 cup Cheese Sauce (page 199)

1 (12-ounce) jar marinated artichoke hearts, drained and quartered

2 tablespoons Plant-Based Parmesan (page 27)

¼ cup minced fresh basil

Per Serving Calories: 728; Total Carbohydrates: 38g; Sugar: 3g; Total Fat: 61g; Saturated Fat: 8g; Sodium: 806mg; Protein: 15g; Fiber: 6g

1. Preheat the oven to 425°F.

2. Coat a large pizza pan with 1 tablespoon of oil and sprinkle with the cornmeal.

3. Stretch the pizza dough and place it in the pan.

4. Par-bake the crust according to the package instructions, about 10 minutes.

5. Meanwhile, in a small skillet over medium heat, heat the remaining 1 tablespoon of oil. Cook the leek with a pinch salt for 5 minutes.

6. Remove the par-baked pizza crust from the oven. Spread the spinach-basil pesto over the pizza. Top with the cheese sauce. Scatter the artichoke hearts and cooked leek over the pizza.

7. Bake for 10 minutes. Allow to rest for 10 minutes before sprinkling with the plant-based Parmesan and basil.

INGREDIENT TIP: To make this dish gluten-free, use a gluten-free pizza dough.

SUBSTITUTION TIP: This pizza can also be made with Tofu Ricotta (page 29) in lieu of the pesto for a nut-free version.

SWEET POTATO NACHOS WITH BARBECUED TEMPEH

Gluten-Free, Make Egg-Free, Make Vegan Nut-Free, Vegetarian

SERVES 4

PREP TIME: 10 minutes COOK TIME: 45 minutes

In this inventive treat, crisp and chewy roasted sweet potatoes are topped with barbecued tempeh and a spicy coleslaw that's to die for! Tempeh is fermented, cooked soybeans and has a nutty, complex flavor and crumbly, chewy texture that works really well in this recipe. The balance of flavors and textures gets me every time.

3 sweet potatoes, unpeeled

3 tablespoons canola oil, divided

Sea salt

1 (8-ounce) package tempeh

1 cup barbecue sauce

2 tablespoons mayonnaise

2 tablespoons freshly squeezed lemon juice

1 teaspoon sugar

½ teaspoon Dijon mustard

1 teaspoon ground cumin

4 cups shredded cabbage

1 Granny Smith apple, julienned

½ red onion, thinly sliced

Per Serving Calories: 517; Total Carbohydrates: 76g; Sugar: 27g; Total Fat: 20g; Saturated Fat: 3g; Sodium: 849mg; Protein: 14g; Fiber: 9g

1. Preheat the oven to 400°F. Line a sheet pan with parchment paper.

2. Slice the sweet potatoes lengthwise into ¼-inch-thick pieces and put them on the sheet pan. Pour 2 tablespoons of oil over the sweet potatoes and toss to coat. Season lightly with salt and shake the pan so the potatoes are in a single layer.

3. Roast for 40 minutes, or until the bottoms of the sweet potatoes are caramelized.

4. Meanwhile, heat the remaining 1 tablespoon of oil in a large skillet over medium heat. Crumble the tempeh into the skillet, and sauté until browned, 3 to 4 minutes. Add the barbecue sauce and cook until just heated through.

5. In a medium bowl, whisk together the mayonnaise, lemon juice, sugar, mustard, and cumin. Add the cabbage, apple, and onion, and toss to coat thoroughly.

6. Divide the sweet potatoes between individual plates. Top with the tempeh and then the coleslaw.

SUBSTITUTION TIP: To make this vegan and egg-free, use a vegan mayonnaise.

MAC 'N' CHEESE

Egg-Free, Gluten-Free, Vegan

SERVES 4

PREP TIME: 5 minutes   COOK TIME: 15 minutes

I tried multiple versions of macaroni and cheese before settling on one that I absolutely loved. The simplest option turned out to be the best! Its inspiration came from the book *Vegan Cooking for Carnivores*, which recommends using a dairy-free cheese. It seems like such an obvious solution, but if you've ever tried dairy-free cheeses, you know how finicky they can be! Fortunately, they work beautifully in this saucy noodle dish.

12 ounces red lentil penne pasta

1 tablespoon Better than Bouillon Vegetable Base

2 tablespoons dairy-free butter, such as Earth Balance Buttery Spread

8 ounces dairy-free cheese such as Follow Your Heart Cheddar Gourmet Shreds

1 cup plain Plain Nut Milk (page 20) made with almonds

Per Serving Calories: 548; Total Carbohydrates: 71g; Sugar: 5g; Total Fat: 24g; Saturated Fat: 8g; Sodium: 982mg; Protein: 16g; Fiber: 7g

1. Bring a large pot of salted water to a boil, and cook the pasta according to the package instructions, about 10 minutes.

2. Drain the pasta, reserving 1 cup of the cooking liquid.

3. Return the reserved cooking liquid to the pot, and whisk in the vegetable base and dairy-free butter.

4. Stir in the dairy-free cheese shreds and almond milk.

5. Return the pasta to the pot and stir until thick, about 2 minutes.

   COOKING TIP: If you cannot find lentil pasta, whole-wheat pasta is just fine, but I like the added protein, fiber, and texture of the lentil penne. You can find it at Trader Joe's and in health food stores.

LASAGNA

Egg-Free, Make Gluten-Free, Nut-Free, Vegan

SERVES 4

PREP TIME: 10 minutes   COOK TIME: 50 minutes

This creamy, comforting, one-pan dinner is everything I missed after going dairy-free. It has become an almost weekly staple in our house because it is so easy to throw together ahead of time and tastes so good. Actually, much like dairy lasagna, it works even better if you make it ahead of time to give the lasagna noodles time to soak up the tomato sauce. Pair it with a side salad, and it easily feeds a family of four.

4 cups Pomodoro Sauce (page 195) or good-quality store-bought marinara sauce, divided

10 ounces no-boil lasagna noodles

1 recipe Tofu Ricotta (page 29)

½ cup roughly chopped fresh basil, divided

2 tablespoons Plant-Based Parmesan (page 27)

Per Serving Calories: 525; Total Carbohydrates: 64g; Sugar: 9g; Total Fat: 22g; Saturated Fat: 3g; Sodium: 995mg; Protein: 22g; Fiber: 3g

1. Preheat the oven to 375°F.

2. Spread 1 cup of sauce in the bottom of an 8-by-11-inch baking dish.

3. Top with 3 lasagna noodles and then cover with 1 cup of sauce. Spread half of the tofu ricotta over the lasagna noodles. It will be a fairly thin layer. Sprinkle with ¼ cup of basil.

4. Repeat the previous step, finishing with lasagna noodles.

5. Top the noodles with the remaining 1 cup of sauce. Sprinkle with the plant-based Parmesan. Cover with aluminum foil and bake for 40 minutes. Remove the foil and continue baking for another 10 minutes.

SUBSTITUTION TIP: I make a gluten-free version of this lasagna with brown rice noodles. My favorite brand is DeBoles.

CHIPOTLE SWEET POTATO QUESADILLAS

Allergen-Free, Egg-Free, Gluten-Free, Nut-Free, Vegan

SERVES 4

PREP TIME: 5 minutes   COOK TIME: 10 minutes

I didn't think a quesadilla without cheese was possible until I tried these. The spicy creaminess of the Sweet Potato Hummus is, dare I say, better than cheese. These open-faced quesadillas make a quick and easy lunch with their satisfying toppings of black beans, guacamole, and lettuce.

2 cups Sweet Potato Hummus (page 72)

8 corn tortillas

1 (15-ounce) can black beans, rinsed and drained

1 cup guacamole

1 cup Dairy-Free Sour Cream (page 192), or store-bought

1 cup shredded lettuce

Per Serving Calories: 488; Total Carbohydrates: 70g; Sugar: 7g; Total Fat: 17g; Saturated Fat: 9g; Sodium: 749mg; Protein: 18g; Fiber: 16g

1. Preheat the oven to 375°F.

2. Spread ¼ cup of sweet potato hummus onto 4 tortillas. Sprinkle each with about 2 tablespoons of black beans. Top each with the remaining tortillas.

3. Place the tortillas on a sheet pan and bake for 10 minutes.

4. Top with 1 tablespoon each of guacamole, sour cream, and shredded lettuce.

SERVING TIP: These can also be rolled into taquitos. Arrange the sweet potato hummus and black beans on one side of each tortilla and roll into a tight cylinder. Brush the taquitos lightly with canola oil and bake for 15 minutes or until lightly browned. Use the guacamole and sour cream for dipping and omit the lettuce.

CHILAQUILES VERDES

Gluten-Free, Vegetarian

SERVES 4

PREP TIME: 10 minutes   COOK TIME: 25 minutes

This vegetarian recipe is one of my favorite savory dishes featuring eggs. The tangy salsa verde, crunchy tostada shells, and tender roasted vegetables play off one another and create a powerful punch of flavors and textures.

2 zucchini, diced

2 red bell peppers, cored and diced

1 red onion, halved and thinly sliced

4 tablespoons canola oil, divided

Sea salt

Freshly ground black pepper

4 eggs

12 tostada shells

1¼ cups Basic Nut Cheese (page 28)

2 cups salsa verde

Per Serving Calories: 739; Total Carbohydrates: 66g; Sugar: 4g; Total Fat: 49g; Saturated Fat: 11g; Sodium: 1219mg; Protein: 18g; Fiber: 6g

1. Preheat the oven to 400°F.

2. Spread out the zucchini, bell peppers, and onion on a sheet pan, and drizzle with 3 tablespoons of oil. Toss gently to coat. Season generously with salt and pepper. Give the pan a shake so the vegetables are in an even layer, and roast for 25 minutes, until caramelized and soft.

3. In a large skillet over medium-high heat, heat the remaining 1 tablespoon of oil. Gently crack the eggs into the skillet without breaking the yolks. Fry the eggs until the whites are set and the yolks are still runny.

4. To serve, top one tostada shell with a spoonful of roasted vegetables, a spoonful of nut cheese, and a drizzle of salsa verde. Top with a second tostada shell, vegetables, nut cheese, and salsa verde. Finish by topping with a third tostada shell, a drizzle of salsa, and one fried egg. Repeat with the remaining ingredients to prepare the other servings. Serve immediately.

SUBSTITUTION TIP: Tostada shells are available in the Mexican foods section of the grocery store. Corn chips can also be used for a more deconstructed presentation.

TORTILLA ESPAÑOLA

Gluten-Free, Nut-Free

SERVES 4

PREP TIME: 5 minutes COOK TIME: 25 minutes

This simple supper has nothing to do with tortillas in the traditional sense. In Spain, tortilla is a ubiquitous tapa made with eggs, potatoes, and onions. I always seem to have these ingredients on hand, so it's a good choice if I haven't planned dinner and need something quick and easy.

2 tablespoons extra-virgin olive oil

2 medium potatoes, thinly sliced

1 yellow onion, thinly sliced

Pinch sea salt

8 eggs, whisked

Per Serving Calories: 270; Total Carbohydrates: 20g; Sugar: 3g; Total Fat: 16g; Saturated Fat: 4g; Sodium: 189mg; Protein: 13g; Fiber: 3g

1. Preheat the oven to 400°F.

2. In a large, deep, oven-safe skillet over medium heat, heat the oil. Add the potatoes, onion, and a generous pinch salt. Cook, stirring occasionally, until gently browned and nearly soft, about 15 minutes.

3. Pour in the eggs. Continue cooking, without stirring, for 5 minutes. Transfer the skillet to the oven for 5 minutes, or until the eggs are set.

4. Cut into wedges to serve.

   SERVING TIP: Tortilla is often served with a red pepper aioli. Use the Aioli (page 191), and stir in 1 tablespoon of adobo sauce or 2 teaspoons of smoked paprika. Alternatively, mix ½ cup of mayonnaise with 1 teaspoon of smoked paprika and 1 tablespoon of freshly squeezed lemon juice.

POTATO GNOCCHI POMODORO

Make Gluten-Free, Nut-Free, Vegetarian

SERVES 4

PREP TIME: 15 minutes   COOK TIME: 20 minutes

Gnocchi is often made with ricotta cheese and Parmesan. This version omits the dairy but keeps the lovely texture and flavor of the dumplings. You really don't need any fancy rolling tools for producing the classic ridged texture; a fork will do just fine. Or, if you prefer a smooth dumpling, like I do, just skip the extra step.

2 pounds russet potatoes, quartered

2 egg yolks

½ teaspoon sea salt

½ cup all-purpose flour or gluten-free flour blend

2 cups Pomodoro Sauce (page 195) or good-quality store-bought marinara sauce

2 tablespoons thinly sliced fresh basil

Per Serving Calories: 276; Total Carbohydrates: 53g; Sugar: 6g; Total Fat: 4g; Saturated Fat: 1g; Sodium: 522mg; Protein: 7g; Fiber: 7g

1. Put the potatoes in a steamer basket set over simmering water. Steam for 15 minutes, or until fork-tender. Allow the potatoes to cool briefly and then mash or press them through a potato ricer.

2. Once the potatoes have cooled enough to handle, stir in the egg yolks, salt, and flour. Mix until just blended. Divide the mixture into 8 portions.

3. On a lightly floured work surface, roll each ball into a long rope, about ¾ inch in diameter. Using a sharp knife or a pasta cutter, cut the rope into 1-inch long sections.

4. Repeat with the remaining dough.

5. Bring a very large pot of salted water to a gentle boil.

6. In a separate pot, bring the sauce to a simmer.

7. Place the gnocchi in the water. When the gnocchi rise to the surface, set a timer for 2 minutes. Use a spider or small mesh strainer to remove the gnocchi from the water, and immediately transfer to the sauce to simmer for 1 minute.

8. Serve garnished with the basil.

    COOKING TIP: Make sure that the water for boiling the gnocchi is not boiling vigorously, which would break up the gnocchi.

SPINACH AND BLACK BEAN ENCHILADAS

Egg-Free, Gluten-Free, Nut-Free, Vegan

SERVES 4

PREP TIME: 15 minutes   COOK TIME: 35 minutes

A similar version of these creamy enchiladas appeared in my first cookbook, *Modern Family Table*, which came out before I went dairy-free. They were a distant memory until I thought to recreate them with dairy-free cream cheese. I'm so happy to have them back in my life. The fragrant cumin and smoked paprika permeate the creamy filling that's packed with vegetables.

1 tablespoon canola oil

1 small yellow onion, diced

4 garlic cloves, minced

Pinch red pepper flakes

1 tablespoon ground cumin

1 teaspoon smoked paprika

8 cups roughly chopped spinach

1 (15-ounce) can black beans

8 ounces dairy-free cream cheese

1 (15-ounce) can red enchilada sauce

12 corn tortillas or 8 flour tortillas

¼ cup minced red onion

¼ cup minced fresh cilantro

1 avocado, diced

1 lime, cut into wedges, for serving

Per Serving Calories: 512; Total Carbohydrates: 58g; Sugar: 4g; Total Fat: 26g; Saturated Fat: 7g; Sodium: 802mg; Protein: 15g; Fiber: 18g

1. Preheat the oven to 375°F.

2. In a large skillet over medium heat, heat the oil. Add the onion and garlic, and cook until soft, about 5 minutes.

3. Add the red pepper flakes, cumin, and paprika, and cook for 1 minute.

4. Add the spinach, and cook until just wilted.

5. Stir in the black beans and dairy-free cream cheese, and cook for 2 minutes, until the cream cheese has melted into the filling.

6. Spread a ½ cup of enchilada sauce over the bottom of an 8-by-10-inch baking dish. Divide the filling between the tortillas, rolling each into a cylinder and placing in the baking dish.

7. Pour the remaining enchilada sauce over the tortillas. Bake for 25 minutes.

8. Sprinkle the onion, cilantro, and avocado over the enchiladas before serving. Garnish with the lime wedges.

COOKING TIP: Corn tortillas are much easier to roll if you heat them individually for 10 to 12 seconds in the microwave.

CREAMY POLENTA VEGETABLE BAKE

Egg-Free, Gluten-Free, Nut-Free, Vegan

SERVES 4

PREP TIME: 5 minutes COOK TIME: 1 hour

Polenta is usually a labor-intensive dish, but this baked polenta lets the oven do all the work. Even better, the vegetables flavor the polenta from the inside out. Since most polenta recipes call for Parmesan or cream, this version uses dairy-free cream cheese for a nice pop of creamy flavor.

1 tablespoon canola oil, plus more for coating the dish

1 small zucchini, thinly sliced

2 cups mushrooms, halved

2 tomatoes, thinly sliced

1 teaspoon minced fresh thyme leaves

1 teaspoon minced fresh rosemary leaves

8 cups vegetable broth

12 ounces polenta

¼ teaspoon sea salt

8 ounces dairy-free cream cheese, cut into pieces

Per Serving Calories: 381; Total Carbohydrates: 27g; Sugar: 7g; Total Fat: 23g; Saturated Fat: 7g; Sodium: 1884mg; Protein: 18g; Fiber: 7g

1. Preheat the oven to 375°F. Coat the interior of a 3-quart casserole dish with oil.

2. In a bowl, mix the zucchini, mushrooms, tomatoes, thyme, and rosemary. Season with the oil. Spread half of the vegetables in the casserole dish.

3. In a large pot, bring the broth to a simmer. Slowly pour in the polenta. Simmer for 5 minutes. Stir in the salt and dairy-free cream cheese, leaving large pieces of cream cheese intact.

4. Spread the polenta into the baking dish, and top with the remaining vegetables.

5. Cover the dish with aluminum foil, and bake for 55 minutes.

COOKING TIP: Unlike traditional cream cheese, dairy-free cream cheese isn't easily cut with a knife. Think of the cutting step more like scooping it into several small spoonfuls. The goal here is to keep the individual chunks of cream cheese from disintegrating into the polenta.

VEGETABLE GARDEN CHILI

Egg-Free, Gluten-Free, Make Allergen-Free, Nut-Free, Vegan

SERVES 4

PREP TIME: 10 minutes COOK TIME: 30 minutes

Mushrooms bring a delicious meaty flavor and texture to this vegan chili. I've been making it the exact same way since my friend Lynn shared her recipe with me 10 years ago. It might seem annoying to use a separate pan to brown the mushrooms, but the distinctive flavor is really worth it. That said, you can also skip the browning step and simply add them to the primary pot.

1 tablespoon canola oil

1 yellow onion, diced

2 carrots, diced

2 celery stalks, finely diced

2 tablespoons dairy-free butter, such as Earth Balance Buttery Spread

2 cups sliced button mushrooms

4 garlic cloves, minced

2 (15-ounce) cans chili beans, drained

2 (15-ounce) cans fire-roasted diced tomatoes

1 tablespoon ground cumin

1 tablespoon smoked paprika

½ teaspoon cayenne pepper

Sea salt

Freshly ground black pepper

1 tablespoon freshly squeezed lime juice

2 avocados, thinly sliced, for serving

½ cup Dairy-Free Sour Cream (page 192) or store-bought for serving

Per Serving Calories: 539; Total Carbohydrates: 47g; Sugar: 11g; Total Fat: 35g; Saturated Fat: 11g; Sodium: 533mg; Protein: 14g; Fiber: 22g

1. In a large pot over medium heat, heat the oil. Add the onion, carrots, and celery, and cook, stirring occasionally, until beginning to soften, about 5 minutes.

2. In a large skillet over high heat, melt the dairy-free butter. Add the mushrooms, and cook for 3 minutes on each side, until well browned. Transfer them to the primary pot.

3. Add the garlic and cook for 30 seconds.

4. Add the beans, tomatoes, cumin, paprika, and cayenne. Season with salt and pepper, and simmer uncovered for 20 minutes. Stir in the lime juice.

5. To serve, garnish with the avocado slices and dairy-free sour cream.

COOKING TIP: For an extra layer of complexity, grate about ½ teaspoon of extra-dark chocolate into the chili just before serving.

FRIED PLANTAIN, BLACK BEAN, AND COLLARD BOWLS

Allergen-Free, Egg-Free, Gluten-Free, Nut-Free, Vegan

SERVES 4

PREP TIME: 5 minutes COOK TIME: 10 minutes

This hearty and tasty meatless dish takes things in a different direction. Here I use plantains, which look like bananas but have a firmer texture and are starchier, with only a hint of sweetness. Think of them the same way you would potatoes, sweet potatoes, or any other starch.

1 (15-ounce) can black beans, drained but not rinsed

1 chipotle pepper in adobo, minced

1 teaspoon adobo sauce

3 tablespoons canola oil, divided

2 barely ripe plantains, cut into ½-inch-thick circles

Sea salt

1 bunch collard greens, ribbed, cut into very thin ribbons

Freshly ground black pepper

2 limes, for serving

Per Serving Calories: 337; Total Carbohydrates: 53g; Sugar: 14g; Total Fat: 12g; Saturated Fat: 1g; Sodium: 77mg; Protein: 11g; Fiber: 12g

1. In a small saucepan over medium-high heat, heat the black beans, chipotle, and adobo sauce until hot, about 2 minutes.

2. In a large skillet over medium-high heat, heat 2 tablespoons of oil. When it is hot, fry the plantains for about 4 minutes on each side, until deeply browned. Divide between four serving dishes. Season with salt.

3. In the same skillet, heat the remaining 1 tablespoon of oil. Add the collard greens, and sauté until they are just wilted and bright green, about 2 minutes. Divide between the serving dishes. Season with salt and pepper.

4. Divide the black beans between the serving dishes, and season with a generous squeeze of lime juice.

INGREDIENT TIP: Make sure to choose plantains that are still a little bit green for a firmer texture.

CRISPY ROASTED TOFU WITH GREEN BEANS

Egg-Free, Gluten-Free, Nut-Free, Vegan

SERVES 4

PREP TIME: 10 minutes COOK TIME: 25 minutes

Sweet hoisin, tangy lime juice, and spicy garlic and red pepper flakes bring everyday tofu and green beans to life. This method for preparing tofu is new to me. For many years, I seared it in oil on the stove top. But it almost always stuck to the pan. Baking it produces a perfectly crisp exterior and chewy middle—who knew? Serve with steamed white rice.

¼ cup low-sodium soy sauce

2 tablespoons freshly squeezed lime juice

2 tablespoons hoisin sauce

1 (14-ounce) package tofu, pressed and cut into ¾-inch pieces

1 tablespoon cornstarch

2 tablespoons canola oil, divided

10 ounces green beans, trimmed

2 teaspoons minced garlic

2 teaspoons minced ginger

Pinch red pepper flakes

Per Serving Calories: 191; Total Carbohydrates: 15g; Sugar: 5g; Total Fat: 12g; Saturated Fat: 2g; Sodium: 1026mg; Protein: 11g; Fiber: 4g

1. Preheat the oven to 400°F. Line a sheet pan with parchment paper.

2. In a small jar, combine the soy sauce, lime juice, and hoisin sauce. Cover tightly with a lid, and shake vigorously. Set aside.

3. Place the tofu in a bowl, and add the cornstarch. Toss gently to coat the tofu pieces in the starch. Drizzle 1 tablespoon of oil over the tofu, and again toss gently to coat. Spread the tofu out on the sheet pan. Bake for 15 to 17 minutes or until the tofu is golden and crispy.

4. Meanwhile, in a large skillet over medium-high heat, heat the remaining 1 tablespoon of oil. Add the green beans, and sauté until crisp tender, 5 to 7 minutes.

5. Add the garlic, ginger, and red pepper flakes to the skillet, and cook until fragrant, about 30 seconds.

6. Remove the skillet from the heat, and add the cooked tofu and soy sauce mixture. Toss everything gently to coat. Serve immediately.

INGREDIENT TIP: To press the tofu, slice it in half horizontally. Place the tofu between two cutting boards and set it on a countertop or over a sink for the water to drain. Set a heavy object on the top cutting board and press for up to 30 minutes.

SPAGHETTI WITH TOFU, SWISS CHARD, AND RED CHILE

Egg-Free, Make Gluten-Free, Nut-Free, Vegan

SERVES 4

PREP TIME: 10 minutes COOK TIME: 30 minutes

This recipe came together as a happy accident. I was wandering through my garden and noticed how beautiful the Swiss chard looked. I pulled together ingredients I had on hand to give this dish a subtle spice from red pepper flakes, earthy minerality from the Swiss chard, and a tangy bite from pickled raisins. Somehow, it just worked, and now the vegan dish is on the menu regularly.

¼ cup raisins

¼ cup red wine vinegar

1 (14-ounce) package tofu, pressed and cut into ¾-inch pieces

1 tablespoon cornstarch

3 tablespoons extra-virgin olive oil, divided

12 ounces spaghetti noodles or gluten-free pasta

1 teaspoon minced garlic

Pinch red pepper flakes

1 bunch Swiss chard, leaves cut into thin ribbons, ribs diced

Sea salt

Freshly ground black pepper

Per Serving Calories: 523; Total Carbohydrates: 76g; Sugar: 9g; Total Fat: 16g; Saturated Fat: 3g; Sodium: 155mg; Protein: 20g; Fiber: 5g

1. Preheat the oven to 400°F. Line a sheet pan with parchment paper.

2. Combine the raisins and vinegar in a small bowl. Set aside.

3. In a bowl, gently toss the tofu in the cornstarch. Drizzle 1 tablespoon of oil over the tofu, and again toss gently to coat. Spread the tofu out on the sheet pan. Bake for 15 to 17 minutes, or until the tofu is golden and crispy.

4. Meanwhile, bring a large pot of salted water to a boil. Cook the pasta according to the package instructions, about 10 minutes.

5. While the pasta is cooking, in a large skillet, heat the remaining 2 tablespoons of oil. Add the garlic and red pepper flakes, and cook until fragrant, about 30 seconds.

6. Add the Swiss chard and cook, stirring occasionally, until just wilted, about 2 minutes.

7. When the pasta has finished cooking, drain it, reserving about ½ cup of the cooking liquid. Transfer the pasta directly to the skillet with the chard, and add just enough cooking liquid to prevent the pasta from sticking.

8. Drain the raisins, reserving about 1 tablespoon of vinegar. Add them both to the pasta, along with the tofu. Season with salt and pepper, give everything a good toss, and serve immediately.

COOKING TIP: I use gluten-free brown rice spaghetti noodles when I prepare this recipe. The brown rice makes the pasta cooking water especially starchy, which brings the pan sauce together nicely.

ROASTED CAULIFLOWER FETTUCINE

Egg-Free, Make Allergen-Free, Make Gluten-Free, Make Nut-Free, Vegan

SERVES 4

PREP TIME: 5 minutes COOK TIME: 45 minutes

I adore roasted cauliflower as an appetizer on its own or over fettucine for a complete meal. The pine nuts are optional, but their salty nuttiness resembles Parmesan and brings a lot to this Sicilian pasta dish.

1 head cauliflower, broken into florets

4 garlic cloves, minced

¼ cup minced fresh parsley

1 teaspoon lemon zest

4 tablespoons extra-virgin olive oil, divided

Sea salt

Freshly ground black pepper

16 ounces fettucine or gluten-free pasta

2 tablespoons red wine vinegar

¼ cup roughly chopped toasted pine nuts (optional)

Per Serving Calories: 572; Total Carbohydrates: 81g; Sugar: 5g; Total Fat: 21g; Saturated Fat: 3g; Sodium: 88mg; Protein: 16g; Fiber: 5g

1. Preheat the oven to 400°F. Line a sheet pan with parchment paper.

2. In a large bowl, mix together the cauliflower, garlic, parsley, and lemon zest. Drizzle with 2 tablespoons of oil, and season generously with salt and pepper. Spread the cauliflower out on the sheet pan and roast for 40 to 45 minutes or until the cauliflower is tender and caramelized.

3. Bring a large pot of salted water to a boil. Cook the pasta according to the package directions. Drain in a colander.

4. Transfer the cooked pasta to a serving dish, add the cauliflower, and toss gently to mix. Drizzle with the remaining 2 tablespoons of oil and the vinegar. Toss again to mix. Top with the pine nuts (if using).

SUBSTITUTION TIP: Use any other roasted vegetable in this recipe if you prefer. I enjoy roasted fennel and red onions with orange zest and basil, too.

GINGER-SOY BROCCOLI PASTA WITH TEMPEH

Egg-Free, Make Gluten-Free, Nut-Free, Vegan

SERVES 4

PREP TIME: 5 minutes COOK TIME: 15 minutes

Somehow my kids love broccoli. I don't know how this happened, but when you find something that works, you just have to go with it. This naturally dairy-free pasta is loaded with two whole heads of broccoli that cook in the pasta cooking liquid, so less cleanup and hassle for me. You don't technically have to cook the tempeh, but giving it a quick sear in hot oil yields a crisp, nutty texture that I can't get enough of.

12 ounces spaghetti noodles or gluten-free pasta

2 heads broccoli, broken into florets

2 tablespoons canola oil

1 (8-ounce) package tempeh, cut into thin 2-inch strips

1 tablespoon freshly squeezed lime juice

¼ cup low-sodium soy sauce

1 teaspoon maple syrup

2 teaspoons toasted sesame oil

1 teaspoon minced garlic

2 teaspoons minced ginger

1 scallion, very thinly sliced on a bias

Per Serving Calories: 585; Total Carbohydrates: 85g; Sugar: 8g; Total Fat: 17g; Saturated Fat: 3g; Sodium: 1010mg; Protein: 28g; Fiber: 8g

1. Bring a large pot of salted water to a boil. Cook the pasta according to the package instructions, about 10 minutes. During the last 3 minutes of cooking time, add the broccoli. Drain in a colander and then transfer to a serving platter.

2. While the pasta cooks, heat the oil in a large skillet over medium-high heat. Sear the tempeh on each side for 2 to 3 minutes, until just browned.

3. In a small jar, combine the lime juice, soy sauce, maple syrup, oil, garlic, and ginger. Seal tightly with a lid, and shake vigorously to combine. Pour over the cooked pasta.

4. Add the broccoli to the pasta and toss to mix. Spread the tempeh pieces over the top, and garnish with the scallion. Serve immediately.

INGREDIENT TIP: To make this dish gluten-free, use gluten-free soy sauce and pasta.

SERVING TIP: The dish can also be served chilled. Simply refrigerate in a covered container until ready to serve.

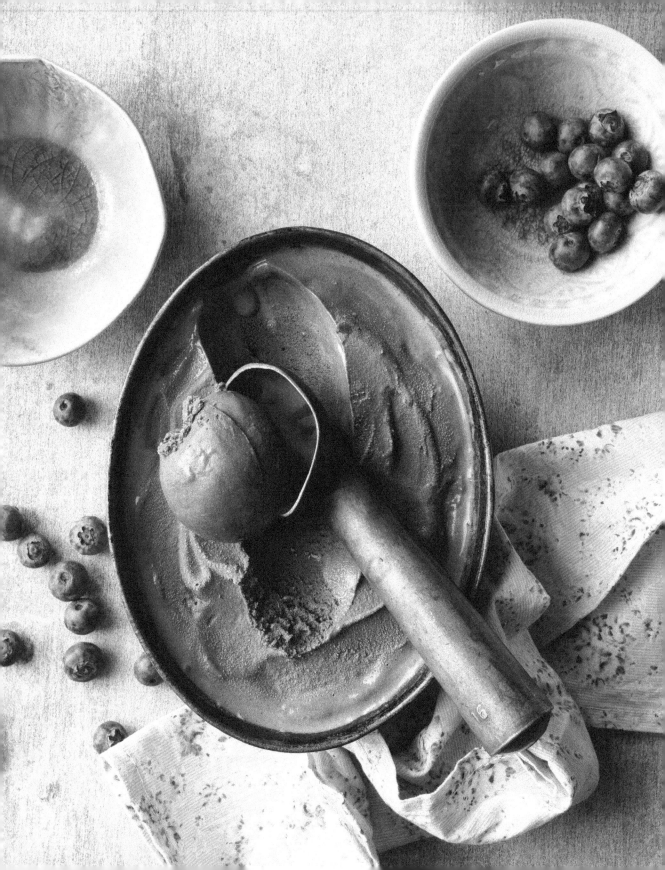

Chapter Eleven

DESSERTS AND SWEET TREATS

Chocolate Ice Cream, page 172

AVOCADO CHOCOLATE PUDDING SNACKS

Egg-Free, Gluten-Free, Make Allergen-Free, Make Nut-Free

SERVES 4

PREP TIME: 5 minutes

Avocados grow prolifically in Santa Barbara, where I live, making this easy, uber-healthy chocolate pudding a regular indulgence. They make a great stand-in for heavy cream because they're dense and creamy, but their flavor is virtually indistinguishable. The quality of the cocoa powder you use matters, so choose an organic, fair-trade cocoa if you can.

2 avocados, pitted and diced

2 bananas, peeled and diced

½ to ¾ cup Plain Nut Milk (page 20) made with almonds, or Rice Milk (page 25)

½ cup cocoa powder

½ cup maple syrup

¼ teaspoon sea salt

Per Serving Calories: 392; Total Carbohydrates: 55g; Sugar: 31g; Total Fat: 22g; Saturated Fat: 5g; Sodium: 163mg; Protein: 5g; Fiber: 12g

1. Place all the ingredients in a blender, starting with ½ cup of nut or rice milk.

2. Purée until smooth, scraping down the sides of the blender a few times to incorporate all of the ingredients, and adding more nut or rice milk as needed. Refrigerate until ready to serve.

INGREDIENT TIP: If you have more ripe avocados than you can possibly use, freeze them. Simply cut them in half, remove the peel and pit and place them cut-side down on a tray lined with parchment paper. Squeeze a small amount of lemon juice over each half and freeze until solid. Transfer to a covered container or resealable plastic bag, and store in the freezer for up to 3 months.

SERVING TIP: Top each pudding with a few slices of banana and some roughly chopped toasted hazelnuts.

BANANA-CASHEW MOUSSE

Egg-Free, Gluten-Free, Vegan

SERVES 4

PREP TIME: 5 minutes, plus 30 minutes to soak

This creamy banana-cashew mousse is a fun afternoon snack, or you can even make it for breakfast. The toasted coconut milk adds complexity and depth, but if you're crunched for time, you can use canned light coconut milk instead.

¾ cup raw cashews, soaked in hot water for at least 30 minutes

2 ripe bananas, sliced, divided

1 cup toasted Coconut Milk (page 24)

¼ cup maple syrup, plus more as needed

2 teaspoons vanilla extract

1 teaspoon ground cinnamon

Pinch sea salt

2 tablespoons coconut oil

Per Serving Calories: 333; Total Carbohydrates: 35g; Sugar: 19g; Total Fat: 19g; Saturated Fat: 8g; Sodium: 64mg; Protein: 6g; Fiber: 3g

1. Rinse and drain the cashews, then combine them with half of the bananas, the coconut milk, maple syrup, vanilla, cinnamon, and salt in a blender. Purée until very smooth.

2. With the motor still running, pour in the oil and blend until thoroughly integrated.

3. Divide the mousse between four serving cups, and top with the remaining sliced bananas.

SERVING TIP: For an extra special dessert, toast ¼ cup of unsweetened coconut, and sprinkle over the mousse as a garnish.

BLUEBERRY CHEESECAKE SNACKS

Egg-Free, Gluten-Free

SERVES 4

PREP TIME: 5 minutes, plus 30 minutes to soak

These adorable pudding cups are naturally raw, vegan, and gluten-free. They're great to make ahead of time and keep in the refrigerator until breakfast, snack time, or dessert—whenever you're craving something smooth, sweet, and creamy.

¾ cup raw cashews, soaked in hot water for at least 30 minutes

½ to 1 cup water

¼ cup maple syrup

1 tablespoon freshly squeezed lemon juice

1 teaspoon vanilla extract

Pinch sea salt

2 tablespoons coconut oil

1 pint fresh blueberries

Per Serving Calories: 294; Total Carbohydrates: 34g; Sugar: 22g; Total Fat: 17g; Saturated Fat: 7g; Sodium: 64mg; Protein: 5g; Fiber: 3g

1. Rinse and drain the cashews, and put them in a blender with ½ cup of water. Blend until smooth, adding only as much water as needed to keep the blender moving.

2. When the cashews are completely smooth, add the maple syrup, lemon juice, vanilla, and salt.

3. With the motor still running, pour in the oil and blend until thoroughly integrated.

4. Divide the mixture between four small ramekins or glass jars. Top each with blueberries. Refrigerate until ready to serve.

SUBSTITUTION TIP: You can use agave nectar in place of maple syrup, but it is 25 percent sweeter, so you may need to use less.

FRENCH SILK CHOCOLATE PIE

Egg-Free, Gluten-Free, Nut-Free

SERVES 12

PREP TIME: 10 minutes COOK TIME: 10 minutes

Silken tofu gives the filling for this pie a smooth, creamy texture, while brewed coffee, vanilla extract, and plenty of dark chocolate bring deep flavor. Compared with dairy-based desserts, this pie is much lower in fat and calories, but it still feels like a decadent treat.

1½ cups crushed graham cracker crumbs

2 tablespoons brown sugar

½ cup dairy-free butter, such as Earth Balance Buttery Spread, melted

11 ounces dairy-free dark chocolate, at least 60 percent cacao

¼ cup brewed coffee

1 (12-ounce) package silken tofu

1 teaspoon vanilla extract

½ teaspoon sea salt

Per Serving Calories: 308; Total Carbohydrates: 30g; Sugar: 16g; Total Fat: 19g; Saturated Fat: 8g; Sodium: 302mg; Protein: 4g; Fiber: 3g

1. Preheat the oven to 375°F.

2. In a food processor, pulse the graham cracker crumbs, sugar, and melted dairy-free butter until finely ground. Pour the mixture into a pie plate, and use the back of a fork to press it down.

3. Bake for 10 minutes, until barely brown. Set aside to cool completely.

4. In a double boiler or a heavy-bottomed pan, melt the chocolate, making sure no water comes in contact with the chocolate. Set aside.

5. In a blender, combine the coffee, tofu, vanilla, and salt. Pour in the melted chocolate, and purée until smooth.

6. Spread the filling into the prepared pie crust. Refrigerate until ready to serve.

INGREDIENT TIP: Read the label of any chocolate you buy to ensure it does not contain dairy.

VANILLA ICE CREAM

Gluten-Free

YIELD: 10 (½-cup) servings

PREP TIME: 5 minutes, plus more to churn

COOK TIME: 10 minutes

This is my go-to vanilla ice cream recipe. I make it often enough that I don't even reach for the recipe anymore, which is not such a feat when you see that it only requires a handful of ingredients. I use both coconut and almond milk because I want the fat of the coconut milk, but I don't want coconut flavor to overpower the ice cream. Half of each seems to be the perfect balance.

2 cups Plain Nut Milk (page 20) made with almonds

1 (15-ounce) can full-fat coconut milk

¾ cup sugar

1 tablespoon vanilla extract

2 tablespoons cornstarch or arrowroot

3 egg yolks

Per Serving Calories: 188; Total Carbohydrates: 20g; Sugar: 17g; Total Fat: 12g; Saturated Fat: 10g; Sodium: 45mg; Protein: 2g; Fiber: 1g

1. In a medium saucepan over medium heat, combine the almond milk, coconut milk, sugar, and vanilla, and cook, whisking constantly, until the sugar dissolves, 2 to 3 minutes.

2. In a medium bowl, whisk together the cornstarch and egg yolks. In a thin stream, pour ½ cup of heated almond milk mixture into the egg yolks, whisking constantly to temper them. Pour the egg yolk mixture into the saucepan, and cook gently, stirring often, until the mixture begins to thicken, 3 to 5 minutes. Do not bring to a simmer or the egg yolks will curdle.

3. Remove the saucepan from the heat, and pour the mixture through a fine mesh sieve into a shallow dish. Cover the top surface of the ice cream base with plastic wrap or parchment paper to prevent the liquid from forming a skin. Refrigerate until thoroughly chilled.

4. Pour the chilled base into the ice cream maker, and follow the manufacturer's instructions.

COOKING TIP: If you don't have an ice cream maker, you can pour the mixture into a chilled bowl and freeze for 30 minutes. Stir with a spatula and freeze again for 15 minutes. Stir every 15 minutes until the ice cream is thick and nearly frozen.

CHOCOLATE ICE CREAM

Gluten-Free

YIELD: 10 (½-cup) servings

PREP TIME: 5 minutes, plus more to churn

COOK TIME: 10 minutes

If you've missed chocolate ice cream since going dairy-free, you're going to love this rich, creamy, dark chocolate dessert. The challenge I find with most store-bought dairy-free ice creams is that they don't use enough chocolate. I hope you'll find this one satisfies your chocolate cravings in every single bite.

2 cups Plain Nut Milk (page 20) made with almonds

1 (15-ounce) can full-fat coconut milk

½ cup sugar

6 ounces dairy-free dark chocolate, broken into pieces

1 tablespoon vanilla extract

¼ teaspoon salt

2 tablespoons cornstarch or arrowroot

3 egg yolks

Per Serving Calories: 265; Total Carbohydrates: 24g; Sugar: 19g; Total Fat: 18g; Saturated Fat: 13g; Sodium: 45mg; Protein: 3g; Fiber: 2g

1. In a medium saucepan over medium heat, combine the almond milk, coconut milk, sugar, chocolate, vanilla, and salt, and cook, whisking constantly, until the chocolate melts and the sugar dissolves, about 5 minutes.

2. In a medium bowl, whisk together the cornstarch and egg yolks. In a thin stream, pour ½ cup of the heated almond milk mixture into the egg yolks, whisking constantly to temper them. Pour the egg yolk mixture into the saucepan and cook gently, stirring often, until the mixture begins to thicken, 3 to 5 minutes. Do not bring to a simmer or the egg yolks will curdle.

3. Remove the pan from the heat, and pour the mixture through a fine mesh sieve into a shallow dish. Cover the top surface of the ice cream base with plastic wrap or parchment paper to prevent the liquid from forming a skin. Refrigerate until thoroughly chilled.

4. Pour the chilled base into the ice cream maker, and follow the manufacturer's instructions.

   SERVING TIP: Serve with fresh blueberries or raspberries for a summertime treat.

MISO-TAHINI ICE CREAM

Allergen-Free, Egg-Free, Gluten-Free, Nut-Free

YIELD: 8 (½-cup) servings

PREP TIME: 5 minutes, plus more to churn

This miso-tahini ice cream tastes like caramel and peanut butter, but is free of both dairy and nuts. And it's a cinch to make—no cooking! Miso might sound like an unusual ingredient for ice cream, but it lends a complex flavor and welcome counterpoint to the sweet, creamy maple syrup and coconut milk.

2 (15-ounce) cans full-fat coconut milk

½ cup maple syrup

1 tablespoon vanilla extract

⅓ cup tahini

1½ tablespoons white miso

Per Serving Calories: 367; Total Carbohydrates: 22g; Sugar: 16g; Total Fat: 31g; Saturated Fat: 23g; Sodium: 149mg; Protein: 5g; Fiber: 3g

1. In a blender, purée all the ingredients until smooth.

2. Refrigerate until thoroughly chilled.

3. Pour the chilled base into the ice cream maker, and follow the manufacturer's instructions.

   SERVING TIP: Top with cacao nibs or a dairy-free chocolate sauce.

SHORTBREAD

Egg-Free, Make Allergen-Free, Make Gluten-Free, Make Nut-Free

SERVES 9

PREP TIME: 5 minutes   COOK TIME: 15 minutes, plus 20 minutes to cool

This flaky, buttery shortbread has just the right amount of sweetness. It's perfect with a midmorning cup of coffee or afternoon tea. Make it extra special by serving with Lemon Curd (page 181) or drizzling with dairy-free chocolate sauce.

2½ cups all-purpose flour or gluten-free flour blend

1 cup dairy-free butter, such as Earth Balance Buttery Spread

½ cup powdered sugar

¼ cup plain Rice Milk (page 25) or Plain Nut Milk (page 20) made with almonds

1 tablespoon vanilla extract

½ teaspoon sea salt

Per Serving Calories: 338; Total Carbohydrates: 34g; Sugar: 7g; Total Fat: 20g; Saturated Fat: 5g; Sodium: 304mg; Protein: 4g; Fiber: 1g

1. Preheat the oven to 400°F. Line an 8-by-8-inch baking dish with parchment paper.

2. In a large bowl, combine all the ingredients, and mix by hand until just blended.

3. Spread the mixture into the baking dish, and smooth out the top with a spatula until flat.

4. Bake for 15 minutes or until the top is golden brown. Allow to cool for 20 minutes before cutting into squares.

COOKING TIP: If you prefer to make this into cookies, roll the dough into a log, wrap in plastic, and refrigerate for 1 hour. Cut into circles and bake for 10 minutes.

CHOCOLATE CHIP COOKIES

Nut-Free

YIELD: 3 dozen small cookies

PREP TIME: 10 minutes   COOK TIME: 10 minutes

Some chocolate chip cookies call for butter, but the problem with butter (besides the fact that it is a dairy product) is that it melts too quickly and contains more water and less fat than vegetable shortening or coconut oil, negatively affecting the texture of the cookie. I prefer baking with coconut oil, or occasionally with vegetable shortening, which works nicely in this recipe.

1 cup vegetable shortening

¾ cup brown sugar

¾ cup white sugar

2 large eggs

1 tablespoon vanilla extract

1 teaspoon sea salt

1 teaspoon baking soda

2¼ cups all-purpose flour or gluten-free flour blend

2 cups dairy-free dark chocolate chips

Per Serving (1 cookie) Calories: 173; Total Carbohydrates: 22g; Sugar: 14g; Total Fat: 10g; Saturated Fat: 4g; Sodium: 91mg; Protein: 2g; Fiber: 0g

1. Preheat the oven to 350°F. Line a sheet pan with parchment paper.

2. In a bowl, beat the shortening, brown sugar, and white sugar with an electric mixer until light and fluffy, about 2 minutes.

3. Add the eggs and vanilla, and beat until thoroughly emulsified.

4. Add the salt, baking soda, and flour, and beat until just blended, using a spatula if necessary to finish incorporating the flour.

5. Fold in the chocolate chips.

6. Scoop the cookie dough into 1-inch balls. Set them on the sheet pan about 2 inches apart, and flatten gently with your hand.

7. Bake for 10 minutes, or until just golden brown around the edges. They should still be soft in the center. Transfer to a cooling rack.

8. Repeat, baking the remaining dough.

INGREDIENT TIP: I like to use a butter-flavored shortening, but it is worth contacting the manufacturer to ensure the product is completely dairy-free.

DOUBLE DARK CHOCOLATE BROWNIES

Make Gluten-Free, Nut-Free

YIELD: 9 brownies

PREP TIME: 5 minutes   COOK TIME: 20 to 22 minutes

In my kitchen, good-quality dark chocolate is as essential as almond milk and eggs. But sometimes I want a dessert that lasts a little longer than a single square of chocolate. Brownies satisfy my cravings, but only when they're the deepest, darkest chocolate.

1 (11-ounce) bag dairy-free dark chocolate chips, preferably 60 percent cacao or more, divided

½ cup coconut oil

4 eggs

½ teaspoon sea salt

½ cup brown sugar

1 tablespoon vanilla extract

1 cup all-purpose flour or gluten-free flour blend

Per Serving Calories: 347; Total Carbohydrates: 31g; Sugar: 18g; Total Fat: 22g; Saturated Fat: 16g; Sodium: 135mg; Protein: 5g; Fiber: 3g

1. Preheat the oven to 350°F. Line the interior of an 8-by-8-inch baking pan with parchment paper.

2. In a double boiler or heavy-bottomed skillet, melt 1 cup of chocolate chips and the oil. Allow to cool.

3. In a separate bowl, beat together the eggs, salt, sugar, and vanilla until smooth, about 1 minute. Add the melted, cooled chocolate mixture. Beat until just integrated.

4. Sift in the flour, and stir until just integrated. Fold in the remaining 3 ounces of chocolate chips.

5. Spread the batter in the prepared pan, and bake for 20 to 22 minutes, until crisp around the edges and just set in the middle.

SERVING TIP: Top the brownies with a generous pinch flaky sea salt as soon as they come out of the oven for a nice contrast of texture and flavor.

CLASSIC WHITE CAKE

Make Gluten-Free, Nut-Free

SERVES 12

PREP TIME: 10 minutes COOK TIME: 20 minutes

Fluffy, moist, and dairy-free, this classic white cake will become your birthday party staple. Fill it with Lemon Curd (page 181) and top with dairy-free Vanilla Frosting (page 182).

¾ cup dairy-free butter, such as Earth Balance Buttery Spread, at room temperature, plus more for greasing the pan

1 cup sugar

¾ cup plain Soy Milk (page 23)

1 teaspoon vanilla extract

2 cups cake flour or gluten-free flour blend

2 teaspoons baking powder

¼ teaspoon sea salt

4 egg whites

Per Serving Calories: 261; Total Carbohydrates: 36g; Sugar: 18g; Total Fat: 12g; Saturated Fat: 3g; Sodium: 169mg; Protein: 4g; Fiber: 1g

1. Preheat the oven to 350°F. Line two 8- or 9-inch cake pans with parchment paper, and grease lightly with dairy-free butter or oil.

2. In a large bowl, beat the dairy-free butter and sugar with a hand mixer until light and fluffy, about 2 minutes.

3. Add the soy milk and vanilla, and beat until just integrated, about 30 seconds.

4. In a medium bowl, sift together the flour, baking powder, and salt. Set aside.

5. In a small bowl, beat the egg whites until voluminous, about 2 minutes.

6. Add one-third of the flour mixture to the large bowl, and beat until just combined. Add one-third of the egg white mixture, and beat until just combined. Repeat until all of the flour and egg white has been incorporated, being careful not to overmix.

7. Divide the batter between the cake pans, and bake for about 20 minutes or until a cake tester comes out clean.

8. Allow the cakes to cool fully before removing from the pans and frosting.

INGREDIENT TIP: For best results, use aluminum-free, double-acting baking powder.

PEACH COBBLER

Egg-Free, Make Gluten-Free

SERVES 9

PREP TIME: 10 minutes COOK TIME: 45 minutes, plus 30 minutes to cool

Peaches are such a special treat, because they're in season for just a short time and quickly fall to the ground. This simple cobbler lets their natural sweetness shine, adding a hint of sugar in the filling and the crusty, delicious, dairy-free biscuit topping.

3 tablespoons dairy-free butter, such as Earth Balance Buttery Spread, divided

8 peaches, cored and sliced

4 tablespoons brown sugar, divided

1 cup all-purpose flour or gluten-free flour blend, plus 2 tablespoons

1½ teaspoons baking powder

¼ teaspoon baking soda

⅔ cup Plain Nut Milk (page 20) made with almonds

1½ teaspoons freshly squeezed lemon juice

Per Serving Calories: 162; Total Carbohydrates: 30g; Sugar: 16g; Total Fat: 5g; Saturated Fat: 1g; Sodium: 88mg; Protein: 3g; Fiber: 3g

1. Preheat the oven to 350°F. Coat the interior of a 2-quart baking dish with 1 tablespoon of dairy-free butter.

2. Place the peaches, 2 tablespoons of sugar, and 2 tablespoons of flour into the baking dish, and toss gently to mix.

3. For the topping, in a food processor, combine the remaining 2 tablespoons of dairy-free butter with the remaining 2 tablespoons of sugar, remaining 1 cup of flour, the baking powder, and baking soda. Pulse until coarsely ground, but pieces of the dairy-free butter remain.

4. Stir in the almond milk and lemon juice until the mixture just comes together.

5. Place spoonfuls of topping over the peaches. Bake for 45 minutes or until the peaches are bubbling and the top is golden brown.

6. Allow to cool for at least 30 minutes before serving.

SERVING TIP: Serve with Vanilla Ice Cream (page 170).

APPLE PIE

Egg-Free, Make Allergen-Free, Make Gluten-Free, Nut-Free

SERVES 8

PREP TIME: 15 minutes   COOK TIME: 45 minutes

My mother-in-law taught me her apple pie recipe before Rich and I were even engaged. We called the pie her "magnum opus," because it rose to impressive heights from the pie dish and was nearly overflowing with crisp, tart apple slices and so much cinnamon it seemed ridiculous. "You can never have too much cinnamon," she says. I tend to agree.

1⅔ cups all-purpose flour or gluten-free flour, plus 2 tablespoons

¼ teaspoon sea salt

1 cup shortening

1 teaspoon freshly squeezed lemon juice

5 to 6 tablespoons ice water

6 to 8 Granny Smith apples, peeled, cored

½ cup brown sugar

1 tablespoon ground cinnamon

¼ teaspoon freshly ground nutmeg

2 tablespoons dairy-free butter, such as Earth Balance Buttery Spread

Per Serving Calories: 461; Total Carbohydrates: 50g; Sugar: 25g; Total Fat: 29g; Saturated Fat: 9g; Sodium: 89mg; Protein: 3g; Fiber: 3g

1. Preheat the oven to 400°F.

2. In a food processor, pulse 1⅔ cups of flour, the salt, and shortening until the mixture has the texture of wet sand.

3. Sprinkle the dough with the lemon juice and just enough water to bind. You may not need to use all the water. Wrap the dough in plastic wrap, and place in the refrigerator.

4. Thinly slice the apples, and toss with the remaining 2 tablespoons of flour, the sugar, cinnamon, and nutmeg.

5. Remove the dough from the refrigerator and divide into two portions. Leave one in the refrigerator while you roll the first.

6. On a lightly floured countertop or on a piece of parchment paper, roll one of the dough portions until it is about 11 inches in circumference. Fold the crust into quarters and carefully transfer it to a 9-inch pie dish. Unfold and gently press it into the pie dish.

continued ☞

7. Place the apples in the crust and top with the dairy-free butter.

8. Roll out the second pie crust like the first, and drape it over the apples. Loosely crimp the edges of the pie in whatever fashion you like. Cut three slits in the top of the pie to vent steam.

9. Bake for 45 minutes, until the pie crust is lightly browned.

INGREDIENT TIP: I like to use the slicing attachment of my food processor to slice the apples. It saves time chopping and helps the apples cook more quickly and form a thicker filling.

LEMON CURD

Gluten-Free, Nut-Free

YIELD: 1 generous cup

PREP TIME: 5 minutes COOK TIME: 10 minutes

You'll find this lemon curd lip-puckering tart! It goes perfectly with biscuits or Shortbread (page 174), and also serves as a tasty cake filling for the Classic White Cake (page 177).

¼ cup dairy-free butter, such as Earth Balance Buttery Spread

⅓ cup freshly squeezed lemon juice

1 teaspoon lemon zest

¼ cup sugar

2 eggs

Per Serving (¼ cup) Calories: 184; Total Carbohydrates: 13g; Sugar: 13g; Total Fat: 13g; Saturated Fat: 4g; Sodium: 145mg; Protein: 3g; Fiber: 0g

1. In a small saucepan over medium-low heat, melt the butter.

2. Whisk in the lemon juice, lemon zest, and sugar, then whisk in the eggs.

3. Cook for 8 to 9 minutes, stirring frequently and being careful not to simmer, until thickened.

INGREDIENT TIP: I'm lucky to have a Meyer lemon tree growing in my backyard, which makes the sweet lemon hybrid a natural choice for this curd. The flavor really is remarkable, so if you can find them in your market, it's worth the splurge.

VANILLA FROSTING

Allergen-Free, Egg-Free, Gluten-Free, Nut-Free

YIELD: 1½ cups

PREP TIME: 5 minutes

Birthdays can be tough on dairy-free kiddos. I remember the first dairy-free birthday cake I made for Brad. At first I felt intimidated making the frosting, but was pleasantly surprised that dairy-free butter and plant-based milks worked like a charm in my traditional frosting recipe. The important thing is to choose a dairy-free butter substitute that you would enjoy slathering on toast. If it doesn't taste good on its own, it's not going to give your frosting a good flavor.

½ cup dairy-free butter, such as Earth Balance Buttery Spread

1 teaspoon vanilla extract

3 cups powdered sugar

Pinch sea salt

4 to 5 teaspoons plain Rice Milk (page 25) or Soy Milk (page 23)

Per Serving (2 tablespoons) Calories: 186;
Total Carbohydrates: 30g; Sugar: 30g; Total Fat: 7g;
Saturated Fat: 2g; Sodium: 94mg; Protein: 0g; Fiber: 0g

1. In a large bowl, beat the dairy-free butter, vanilla, sugar, and salt with a hand mixer until thoroughly blended.

2. Add the rice milk, a teaspoon at a time, until the frosting reaches your desired consistency.

   SUBSTITUTION TIP: For chocolate frosting, add ½ cup unsweetened cocoa powder and increase the plant-based milk by an additional 1 to 2 tablespoons.

COCONUT WHIPPED CREAM

Allergen-Free, Egg-Free, Gluten-Free, Nut-Free

YIELD: 2 cups

PREP TIME: 5 minutes

This whipped cream is simple, easy, and relatively healthy. You can serve it with Apple Pie (page 179), Peach Cobbler (page 178), Double Dark Chocolate Brownies (page 176), or whenever you would normally serve whipped cream.

1 (14-ounce) can coconut cream

½ teaspoon vanilla extract

¼ cup powdered sugar

Per Serving (¼ cup) Calories: 213; Total Carbohydrates: 33g; Sugar: 32g; Total Fat: 9g; Saturated Fat: 9g; Sodium: 20mg; Protein: 1g; Fiber: 0g

1. Refrigerate the coconut cream and a metal mixing bowl overnight. Do not shake the can at any time before or after refrigerating.

2. Carefully open the coconut cream. Scoop off the top layer of cream (about half the can), and transfer it to the chilled bowl. Set aside the remaining liquid for another use (see Ingredient tip).

3. Beat with a hand mixer for 1 minute. Add the vanilla and powdered sugar, and continue beating for another 2 minutes, or until thick and fluffy.

INGREDIENT TIP: If you cannot find coconut cream, use two cans of coconut milk. The remaining liquid from coconut milk or coconut cream can be used for baking or in smoothies.

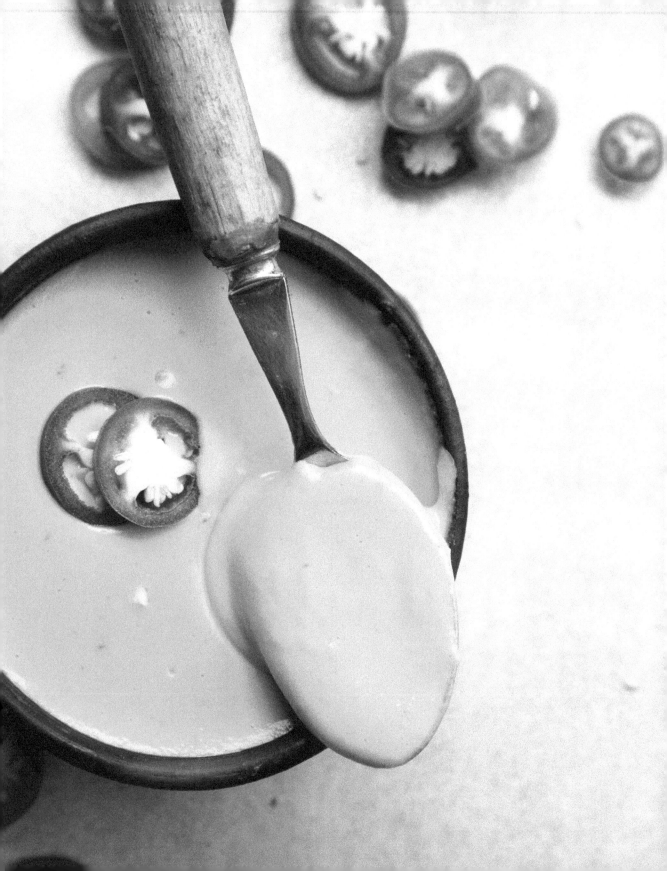

Chapter Twelve

SAUCES, CONDIMENTS, AND DRESSINGS

Nacho Cheese Sauce, page 200

BALSAMIC VINAIGRETTE

Allergen-Free, Egg-Free, Gluten-Free, Nut-Free, Vegan

YIELD: 1 cup

PREP TIME: 5 minutes

In 2012, several earthquakes rocked the region of Italy that produces balsamic vinegar. I was traveling in the country at that time and felt some of the tremors that turned out to be catastrophic to the industry, damaging thousands of gallons of aging vinegar. A few years later, my brother sent me a few small bottles of aged balsamic. Its scarcity made it that much sweeter and more special. Use a good quality balsamic in this recipe for the best flavor.

1 shallot, minced

1 tablespoon fresh basil, minced

⅓ cup balsamic vinegar

⅔ cup extra-virgin olive oil

1 teaspoon maple syrup

Sea salt

Freshly ground black pepper

Per Serving (2 tablespoons) Calories: 154; Total Carbohydrates: 2g; Sugar: 2g; Total Fat: 17g; Saturated Fat: 2g; Sodium: 9mg; Protein: 0g; Fiber: 0g

In a small jar, combine all the ingredients. Cover tightly with a lid, and shake until emulsified.

HONEY DIJON DRESSING

Egg-Free, Gluten-Free, Nut-Free

YIELD: 1 cup

PREP TIME: 5 minutes

Honey and Dijon mustard are both emulsifiers, meaning they integrate the oil and vinegar into a smooth, creamy dressing. They also add a touch of sweetness and spice.

1 shallot, minced

1 small garlic clove, minced

⅓ cup apple cider vinegar

⅔ cup extra-virgin olive oil

1 tablespoon honey

1 teaspoon Dijon mustard

Sea salt

Freshly ground black pepper

Per Serving (2 tablespoons) Calories: 158; Total Carbohydrates: 3g; Sugar: 2g; Total Fat: 17g; Saturated Fat: 2g; Sodium: 9mg; Protein: 0g; Fiber: 0g

In a small jar, combine all the ingredients. Cover tightly with a lid, and shake until emulsified.

RANCH DRESSING

Gluten-Free, Nut-Free, Vegetarian

YIELD: 1 cup

PREP TIME: 5 minutes

Cool, creamy, and just what you crave in ranch, this dressing works great on salads and as a dip for vegetables. Bonus: Unlike the store-bought ranch dressings, this one is free of preservatives and artificial ingredients!

¾ cup mayonnaise

¼ cup Dairy-Free Sour Cream (page 192) or store-bought

2 tablespoons minced fresh parsley

2 tablespoons minced fresh chives

1 tablespoon minced fresh dill

1 teaspoon minced garlic

¼ teaspoon sea salt

¼ teaspoon freshly ground black pepper

¼ cup plain Soy Milk (page 23)

Per Serving (2 tablespoons) Calories: 107; Total Carbohydrates: 7g; Sugar: 2g; Total Fat: 9g; Saturated Fat: 2g; Sodium: 228mg; Protein: 1g; Fiber: 0g

In a bowl, stir together the mayonnaise, sour cream, parsley, chives, dill, garlic, salt, and pepper until well blended. If creating a dip, stop here. To thin it for salad dressing, slowly drizzle in the soy milk and whisk to blend.

INGREDIENT TIP: I like the garlic very finely minced for this recipe, so I use a Microplane grater to get a purée of garlic, which disburses evenly throughout the dressing.

CAESAR DRESSING

Gluten-Free, Nut-Free

YIELD: ¾ cup

PREP TIME: 5 minutes

A good Caesar salad can still be part of your dairy-free life with this awesome Caesar dressing. The flavors are fresh and so much better than the bottled stuff anyway.

2 egg yolks

2 tablespoons freshly squeezed lemon juice

1 teaspoon minced anchovies

1 teaspoon minced garlic

½ teaspoon Dijon mustard

½ teaspoon freshly ground black pepper

¼ teaspoon sea salt

½ cup canola oil

¼ cup olive oil

Per Serving (2 tablespoons) Calories: 260; Total Carbohydrates: 1g; Sugar: 0g; Total Fat: 29g; Saturated Fat: 3g; Sodium: 209mg; Protein: 1g; Fiber: 0g

1. In a medium bowl, stir together the egg yolks, lemon juice, anchovies, garlic, mustard, salt, and pepper.

2. Slowly drizzle in the canola oil and olive oil, whisking constantly until emulsified.

   SUBSTITUTION TIP: To make a vegetarian version, omit the anchovies and increase the sea salt to ½ teaspoon.

GREEN GODDESS DRESSING

Gluten-Free, Nut-Free, Vegetarian

YIELD: 1½ cups

PREP TIME: 5 minutes

Tarragon is an underappreciated herb but it gets its due in this classic salad dressing created in San Francisco in the 1920s. With its variety of greens lending to the name, this dressing is something special. Try it with Bibb lettuce and croutons.

4 scallions, trimmed, roughly chopped

¼ cup fresh basil, roughly chopped

2 tablespoons roughly chopped fresh tarragon

2 tablespoons freshly squeezed lemon juice

2 garlic cloves, smashed

½ cup mayonnaise

½ cup Dairy-Free Sour Cream (page 192) or store-bought

1 teaspoon sea salt

Per Serving (2 tablespoons) Calories: 62;
Total Carbohydrates: 4g; Sugar: 2g; Total Fat: 5g;
Saturated Fat: 2g; Sodium: 237mg; Protein: 1g; Fiber: 0g

Place all of the ingredients in a blender, and purée until smooth.

INGREDIENT TIP: Basil and tarragon are easy to grow in windowsill gardens. I like to grow them so I'll always have some on hand. Unlike with packaged herbs, none goes to waste because I only pick what I need.

AIOLI

Gluten-Free, Nut-Free, Vegetarian

YIELD: ½ cup

PREP TIME: 5 minutes

I love this naturally dairy-free sauce. It's creamy and thick, and everything I'm craving on a dairy-free diet. Aioli is delicious as it is, or you can kick up the heat and whisk in a teaspoon of adobo sauce and drizzle it over Tortilla Española (page 153) or offer as a dip for Sweet Potato Corn Cakes (page 78).

1 egg yolk

1 teaspoon freshly squeezed lemon juice

1 small garlic clove, minced

½ cup canola oil

Per Serving (1 tablespoon) Calories: 115; Total Carbohydrates: 0g; Sugar: 0g; Total Fat: 13g; Saturated Fat: 2g; Sodium: 1mg; Protein: 0g; Fiber: 0g

1. In a small bowl, whisk together the egg yolk, lemon juice, and garlic.

2. Slowly drizzle in the oil a few drops at a time, whisking constantly to emulsify, until thick and pale.

3. Store in a covered container in the refrigerator for up to 3 days.

COOKING TIP: Consuming raw egg yolk increases the risk of foodborne illness.

DAIRY-FREE SOUR CREAM

Egg-Free, Gluten-Free, Nut-Free, Vegan

YIELD: 1½ cups

PREP TIME: 5 minutes

I usually keep silken tofu on hand in my cupboard, which makes this dairy-free sour cream easy to whip up at a moment's notice. It's useful for many applications throughout this cookbook and beyond, including Corn Chowder (page 61), Beef Stroganoff (page 123), and Vegetable Garden Chili (page 157).

1 (11-ounce) package silken tofu

2 tablespoons apple cider vinegar

1 tablespoon freshly squeezed lemon juice

½ teaspoon minced fresh garlic

¼ teaspoon sea salt

Per Serving (2 tablespoons) Calories: 17; Total Carbohydrates: 1g; Sugar: 0g; Total Fat: 1g; Saturated Fat: 0g; Sodium: 49mg; Protein: 2g; Fiber: 0g

Place all the ingredients in a blender, and purée until smooth, scraping down the sides as needed.

INGREDIENT TIP: Silken tofu is found in the Asian foods section of the supermarket and is not typically refrigerated.

SPINACH-BASIL PESTO

Egg-Free, Gluten-Free, Vegan

YIELD: 2 cups

PREP TIME: 5 minutes

Most pesto is made with Parmesan cheese. This version uses a touch of nutritional yeast and a generous amount of pine nuts and sea salt instead. You won't even miss the dairy. I love serving it on Creamy Artichoke and Pesto Pizza (page 147).

½ cup extra-virgin olive oil

3 garlic cloves, smashed

2 cups loosely packed fresh spinach

2 cups loosely packed fresh basil

½ cup toasted pine nuts, roughly chopped

1 tablespoon nutritional yeast

1 teaspoon freshly squeezed lemon juice

½ teaspoon sea salt

¼ teaspoon freshly ground black pepper

Per Serving (2 tablespoons) Calories: 89; Total Carbohydrates: 1g; Sugar: 0g; Total Fat: 9g; Saturated Fat: 1g; Sodium: 62mg; Protein: 1g; Fiber: 1g

1. Place all the ingredients into a blender in the order listed.

2. Pulse a few times, then stop the motor, and press down on the spinach and basil with a spatula as needed to make sure the blades are reaching it.

3. Blend until thoroughly integrated but still slightly chunky.

   SUBSTITUTION TIP: You can use kale or arugula in place of the spinach for a slightly different flavor. Kale is a bit sweeter, and arugula has a peppery flavor. You can also use walnuts, cashews, or pecans in place of the pine nuts.

SALSA VERDE

Allergen-Free, Egg-Free, Gluten-Free, Nut-Free, Vegan

YIELD: 2½ cups

PREP TIME: 5 minutes COOK TIME: 30 minutes

This tangy salsa verde is naturally dairy-free and makes a delicious accompaniment to roasted meat. It can also be served over Chilaquiles Verdes (page 152) or simply presented with corn tortilla chips for dipping.

2 cups quartered tomatillos, husked and rinsed (see Ingredient tip)

½ red onion, thinly sliced

2 garlic cloves, unpeeled

1 serrano pepper, quartered lengthwise

2 tablespoons canola oil

Sea salt

2 tablespoons freshly squeezed lime juice

½ cup roughly chopped fresh cilantro

Per Serving (¼ cup) Calories: 34; Total Carbohydrates: 2g; Sugar: 0g; Total Fat: 3g; Saturated Fat: 0g; Sodium: 24mg; Protein: 0g; Fiber: 1g

1. Preheat the oven to 400°F. Line a sheet pan with parchment paper.

2. Spread the tomatillos, onion, garlic, and pepper on the sheet pan. Toss with the oil and season with salt. Roast uncovered for 30 minutes or until the tomatillos are tender. Be watchful not to burn the onion.

3. When cool enough to handle, squeeze the garlic pulp from the skins into a blender. Discard the skins. Add the rest of the vegetable mixture and the lime juice and cilantro to the blender, and purée until mostly smooth.

INGREDIENT TIP: To prepare the tomatillos, remove the rough husks and rinse the fruits in warm water to remove the sticky residue.

POMODORO SAUCE

Allergen-Free, Egg-Free, Gluten-Free, Nut-Free, Vegan

YIELD: 4 cups

PREP TIME: 5 minutes
COOK TIME: 30 to 45 minutes

Its simplicity might lead you to believe that this pomodoro sauce is nothing special, but once you taste it, you'll find that its simplicity is what makes it so great. The flavor of the cooked fresh tomatoes is intense without being overpowering. Use this recipe to make the Deep Dish Veggie Pizza (page 146) and the Potato Gnocchi Pomodoro (page 154).

2 pounds tomatoes, quartered and stemmed

2 tablespoons extra-virgin olive oil

2 teaspoons sea salt

¼ cup minced fresh basil

Per Serving (½ cup) Calories: 51; Total Carbohydrates: 4g; Sugar: 1g; Total Fat: 4g; Saturated Fat: 1g; Sodium: 474mg; Protein: 1g; Fiber: 3g

1. In a large pot over medium-low heat, cook the tomatoes, oil, and salt until the tomatoes are broken down and fragrant, 30 to 45 minutes.

2. Remove from the heat, and stir in the basil.

3. Use an immersion blender to purée the sauce until smooth.

   COOKING TIP: If you don't have an immersion blender, carefully transfer the sauce to a blender. Cover the lid with a towel and vent to allow steam to escape, being careful of spattering.

TZATZIKI

Egg-Free, Gluten-Free, Vegan

YIELD: 3 cups

PREP TIME: 5 minutes

Traditional tzatziki is made with yogurt. This version uses plain almond milk yogurt and sour cream for a similar flavor and texture. I think it's good enough to share. Try it in Meatball Wraps with Tzatziki (page 117).

1 cup minced cucumber

1 cup dairy-free plain yogurt, preferably almond milk yogurt

1 cup Dairy-Free Sour Cream (page 192) or store-bought

1 teaspoon minced garlic

1 tablespoon minced fresh mint

2 tablespoons extra-virgin olive oil

¼ teaspoon sea salt

½ teaspoon freshly ground black pepper

Per Serving (¼ cup) Calories: 97; Total Carbohydrates: 6g; Sugar: 4g; Total Fat: 8g; Saturated Fat: 4g; Sodium: 61mg; Protein: 1g; Fiber: 0g

In a small bowl, mix the cucumber, yogurt, sour cream, garlic, and mint. Slowly drizzle in the oil, whisking constantly. Add the salt and pepper.

INGREDIENT TIP: Read the label on whichever yogurt you choose. Many contain added sugar, which will make the tzatziki too sweet.

WHITE SAUCE

Egg-Free, Make Gluten-Free, Make Nut-Free, Vegan

YIELD: 2 cups

PREP TIME: 5 minutes   COOK TIME: 5 minutes

Dairy-free butter and flour thicken this simple white sauce. I think it's best with pasta or drizzled over pizza. Most white sauce recipes call for white pepper but it doesn't have a pleasant aroma, so I prefer to keep it plain and season the finished dish with freshly ground black pepper.

3 tablespoons dairy-free butter, such as Earth Balance Buttery Spread

3 tablespoons all-purpose flour or gluten-free flour blend

2 cups Plain Nut Milk (page 20) made with almonds, or Soy Milk (page 23)

Sea salt

Per Serving (¼ cup) Calories: 58; Total Carbohydrates: 3g; Sugar: 0g; Total Fat: 5g; Saturated Fat: 1g; Sodium: 118mg; Protein: 1g; Fiber: 0g

1. In a medium saucepan over medium heat, melt the dairy-free butter. Whisk in the flour until no lumps remain. Cook, whisking, for 2 minutes.

2. Add the almond or soy milk all at once, whisking vigorously.

3. Cook until thickened, about 2 minutes. Do not boil. Season with salt.

COOKING TIP: For an Alfredo sauce, add 1 teaspoon of minced garlic and 1 tablespoon of nutritional yeast.

GRAVY

Allergen-Free, Egg-Free, Make Gluten-Free, Nut-Free

YIELD: 2 cups

PREP TIME: 5 minutes COOK TIME: 5 minutes

Good news: Dairy-free butter works just as well as regular butter for making gravy. The important thing is to use the best-quality chicken broth. I like to make broth from roasted chicken bones (see Cooking tip, page 112).

3 tablespoons dairy-free butter, such as Earth Balance Buttery Spread

3 tablespoons all-purpose flour or gluten-free flour blend

2 cups chicken broth

Sea salt

Freshly ground black pepper

Per Serving (¼ cup) Calories: 58; Total Carbohydrates: 3g; Sugar: 0g; Total Fat: 5g; Saturated Fat: 1g; Sodium: 268mg; Protein: 2g; Fiber: 0g

1. In a small saucepan over medium heat, melt the dairy-free butter. Whisk in the flour until no lumps remain. Cook, whisking, for 2 minutes, or longer for a deeper roux.

2. Add the broth all at once, whisking vigorously.

3. Cook until thickened, about 2 minutes. Season with salt and pepper.

   COOKING TIP: Instead of dairy-free butter, you can use pan drippings or chicken fat, also known as "schmaltz."

CHEESE SAUCE

Egg-Free, Gluten-Free, Vegan

YIELD: 1½ cups

PREP TIME: 5 minutes, plus 30 minutes to soak

This sauce works like a charm in Mac 'n' Cheese (page 149), slathered over Creamy Artichoke and Pesto Pizza (page 147), and on baked potatoes. The flavor is pretty strong, so add the nutritional yeast a little bit at a time until it reaches your desired flavor.

1 cup raw cashews

1 cup Plain Nut Milk (page 20) made with almonds

1 tablespoon white miso

1 teaspoon garlic powder

1 teaspoon onion powder

½ teaspoon sea salt

3 to 5 tablespoons nutritional yeast

Per Serving (¼ cup) Calories: 196; Total Carbohydrates: 15g; Sugar: 4g; Total Fat: 12g; Saturated Fat: 2g; Sodium: 301mg; Protein: 11g; Fiber: 2g

1. Soak the cashews in hot water for 30 minutes to soften. Rinse and drain.

2. In a blender, combine the cashews, almond milk, miso, garlic powder, onion powder, and salt. Purée until smooth.

3. Add the nutritional yeast 1 tablespoon at a time, and purée until integrated, scraping down the sides as needed.

SUBSTITUTION TIP: For a soy-free version, omit the miso.

NACHO CHEESE SAUCE

Egg-Free, Gluten-Free, Vegan

YIELD: 1½ cups

PREP TIME: 5 minutes, plus 30 minutes to soak

This sauce features a few extra spices for that nacho essence, making it great for dipping corn tortilla chips or jalapeño slices, or anywhere else you enjoy nacho cheese sauce.

1 cup raw cashews

1 cup Plain Nut Milk (page 20) made with almonds

2 teaspoons garlic powder

1 teaspoon onion powder

1 teaspoon ground turmeric

1 teaspoon smoked paprika

½ teaspoon sea salt

2 tablespoons nutritional yeast

Per Serving Calories: 161; Total Carbohydrates: 11g; Sugar: 1g; Total Fat: 12g; Saturated Fat: 2g; Sodium: 192mg; Protein: 7g; Fiber: 2g

1. Soak the cashews in hot water for 30 minutes to soften. Rinse and drain.

2. In a blender, combine the cashews, almond milk, garlic powder, onion powder, turmeric, smoked paprika, and salt. Purée until smooth.

3. Add the nutritional yeast 1 tablespoon at a time, and purée until integrated, scraping down the sides as needed.

SUBSTITUTION TIP: Instead of cashews, you can use macadamia nuts.

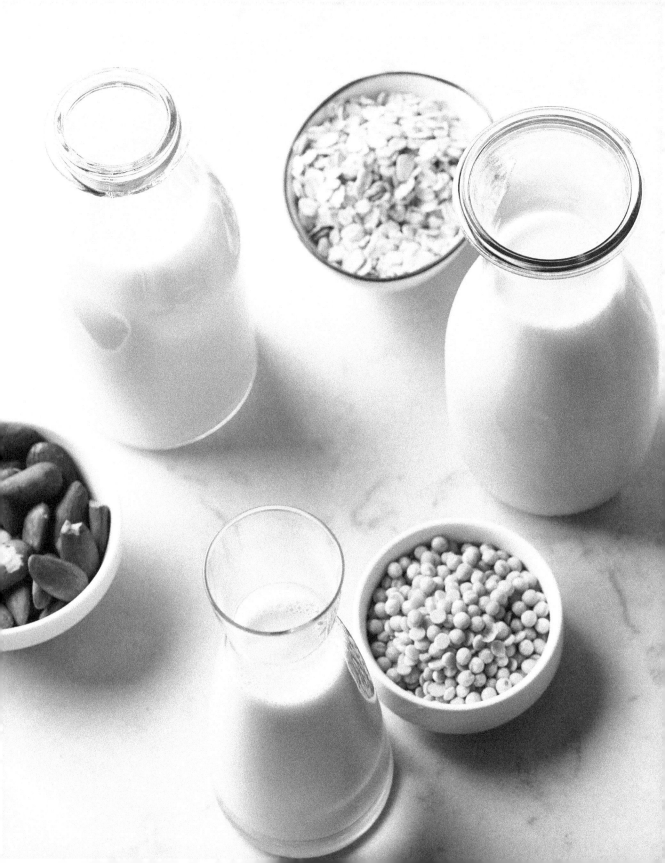

SUGGESTED MENUS

New Year's Eve

Cranberry and Cracked Pepper Cheese Ball
(page 70)

Chicken Cassoulet (page 141)

French Silk Chocolate Pie (page 169)

Easter

Strawberry-Spinach Salad (page 58)

Rosemary Pork Tenderloin with
Plum Sauce (page 110)

Lemon Curd (page 181) with Shortbread
(page 174)

Fourth of July

Coffee-Glazed Steak (page 121)

Tomato, Mint, and Shallot Salad (page 52)

Mashed Potatoes (page 84)

Peach Cobbler (page 178) and Vanilla
Ice Cream (page 170)

Thanksgiving

Bourbon Mashed Sweet Potatoes (page 85)

Sautéed Brussels Sprouts (page 77)

Herb and Garlic Roasted Chicken
(or turkey) (page 128)

Apple Pie (page 179)

Christmas or Hanukkah

Caesar Salad (page 54)

Balsamic Pot Roast (page 120)

Rosemary Roasted Potatoes (page 82)

Shortbread (page 174)

Birthday Parties

Pepperoni, Red Onion, and Cherry Tomato
Pizza (page 106)

Classic White Cake (page 177)

Vanilla Frosting (page 182)

THE DIRTY DOZEN
& THE CLEAN FIFTEEN

A nonprofit and environmental watchdog organization called the Environmental Working Group (EWG) looks at data supplied by the US Department of Agriculture (USDA) and the Food and Drug Administration (FDA) about pesticide residues. Each year it compiles a list of the lowest and highest pesticide loads found in commercial crops. You can use these lists to decide which fruits and vegetables to buy organic to minimize your exposure to pesticides and which produce is considered safe enough to buy conventionally. This does not mean they are pesticide-free, though, so wash these fruits and vegetables thoroughly.

These lists change every year, so make sure you look up the most recent one before you fill your shopping cart. You'll find the most recent lists as well as a guide to pesticides in produce at EWG.org/FoodNews.

THE DIRTY DOZEN*

- Apples
- Celery
- Cherry tomatoes
- Cucumbers
- Grapes
- Nectarines (imported)
- Peaches
- Potatoes
- Snap peas (imported)
- Spinach
- Strawberries
- Sweet bell peppers

* Kale/Collard greens & Hot peppers

THE CLEAN FIFTEEN

- Asparagus
- Avocados
- Cabbage
- Cantaloupes (domestic)
- Cauliflower
- Eggplants
- Grapefruits
- Kiwis
- Mangos
- Onions
- Papayas
- Pineapples
- Sweet corn
- Sweet peas (frozen)
- Sweet potatoes

* In addition to the dirty dozen, the EWG added two produce contaminated with highly toxic organophosphate insecticides.

RESOURCES

Books

Against All Grain: Delectable Paleo Recipes to Eat Well & Feel Great, by Danielle Walker

Babycakes: Vegan, (Mostly) Gluten-Free, and (Mostly) Sugar-Free Recipes from New York's Most Talked-About Bakery, by Erin McKenna

Cast Iron Paleo: 101 One-Pan Recipes for Quick-and-Delicious Meals plus Hassle-free Cleanup, by Pamela Ellgen

Minimalist Baker's Everyday Cooking: 101 Entirely Plant-Based, Mostly Gluten-Free, Easy and Delicious Recipes, by Dana Shultz

The Gluten-Free Cookbook for Families: Healthy Recipes in 30 Minutes or Less, by Pamela Ellgen and Alice Bast

The New Milks: 100-Plus Dairy-Free Recipes for Making and Cooking with Soy, Nut, Seed, Grain, and Coconut Milks, by Dina Cheney

This Cheese Is Nuts: Delicious Vegan Cheese at Home, by Julie Piatt

Vegan Cooking for Carnivores: Over 125 Recipes So Tasty You Won't Miss the Meat, by Roberto Martin

Websites

Go Dairy Free: www.godairyfree.org

Minimalist Baker: www.minimalistbaker.com

Vegan.com: www.vegan.com

REFERENCES

Barnard, Neal. *The Cheese Trap: How Breaking a Surprising Addiction Will Help You Lose Weight, Gain Energy, and Get Healthy.* New York: Grand Central Life and Style, 2017.

Bottom Line, Inc. "What You Eat (or Don't) Eat Affects Your Sleep." Accessed August 5, 2017. http://bottomlineinc.com/health /insomnia/what-you-eat-or-dont-eat-affects -how-you-sleep.

De Biase, Simone G., Sabrina F.C. Fernandes, Reinaldo J. Gianini, and João L.G. Duarte. "Vegetarian Diet and Cholesterol and Triglycerides Levels." *Arquivos Brasileiros de Cardiologia* 88, no. 1 (January 2007).

Food Allergy Research and Education. "Milk Allergy." Accessed July 29, 2017. https://www.foodallergy.org/allergens /milk-allergy.

Gibbons, Ann. "How Europeans Evolved White Skin." *Science Magazine: American Association for the Advancement of Science.* Accessed July 28, 2017. http://www .sciencemag.org/news/2015/04/ how -europeans-evolved-white-skin.

Lifschitz, C., and H. Szajewska. "Cow's Milk Allergy: Evidence-Based Diagnosis and Management for the Practitioner." European Journal of Pediatrics 174 (February 2015): 141–150.

Mu, Q., J. Kirby, C.M. Reilly, and X.M. Luo. "Leaky Gut as a Danger Signal for Autoimmune Diseases." *Frontiers in Immunology* 8 (May 2017): 598.

National Institutes of Health, Office of Dietary Supplements. "Calcium: Fact Sheet for Professionals." Accessed August 10, 2017.

National Institutes of Health, Office of Dietary Supplements. "Vitamin D: Fact Sheet for Professionals." Accessed August 11, 2017.

Physicians Committee for Responsible Medicine. "USDA Panel Backs Doctors' Complaints against Milk Ads." September 22, 2001. http://www.newswise.com //articles/usda-panel-backs-doctors -complaints-against-milk-ads. Accessed August 10, 2017.

Precision Nutrition. "Vitamin D Supplements: Are Yours Helping or Hurting?" Accessed August 11, 2017. http:// www.precisionnutrition.com/stop-vitamin-d.

Simple Vegan Blog. "Homemade Soy Milk." Accessed August 5, 2017. http:// simpleveganblog.com/homemade-soy-milk/

Tai Le, Lap, and Joan Sabaté. "Beyond Meatless, the Health Effects of Vegan Diets: Findings from the Adventist Cohorts." *Nutrients* 6, no. 6 (June 2014): 2131–47.

The Blender Girl 2.0 Simple Tricks and Tips. "Plant-Based Milks." Accessed August 5, 2017. http://healthyblenderrecipes.com /hints_tips/plant_based_milks.

Tokede, O.A., J.M. Gaziano, and L. Djoussé. "Effects of Cocoa Products/Dark Chocolate on Serum Lipids: A Meta-Analysis." European Journal of Clinical Nutrition 65, no. 8 (August 2011): 879–86.

Tonstad, S., K. Stewart, K. Oda, M. Batech, R.P. Herring, and G.E. Fraser. "Vegetarian Diets and Incidence of Diabetes in the Adventist Health Study-2." *Nutrition, Metabolism, and Cardiovascular Disease* 23, no. 4 (April 2013): 292-9.

Vitamin D Council. "How Do I Get the Vitamin D My Body Needs?" Accessed August 8, 2017. https://www .vitamindcouncil.org/about-vitamin-d/how -do-i-get-the-vitamin-d-my-body-needs/.

WebMD. "Confused About Calcium Supplements?" Accessed August 11, 2017. http://www.webmd.com/osteoporosis /calcium-supplements-tips#1.

WebMD. "Find a Vitamin or Supplement: Vitamin D." Accessed August 11, 2017. http://www.webmd.com/vitamins -supplements/ingredientmono-929 -vitamin%20d.aspx?activeingredientid=929.

RECIPE INDEX

INDEX

D

E

V

ACKNOWLEDGMENTS

Special thanks to the amazing team at Callisto Media, especially Meg Ilasco, Patty Consolazio, and the design team, who always makes the books so beautiful. You are a pleasure to work with and bring out the best in me.

Thank you, Brad and Cole, for putting up with my sometimes-unpalatable attempts at mac 'n' cheese, nachos, pizza, and lasagna as I tried to get the recipes just right. You were tough critics, and the book is better for it. Thanks, guys! Let's make some coconut ice cream, okay?

Thank you, Rich, for your willingness to eat a lot of different things all in the name of recipe testing.

Thank you, Mom, for teaching me early that dairy isn't necessarily the perfect food for people.

Thank you especially to all of the vegan and dairy-free chefs who have paved the way toward delicious dairy-free living. To the first person who thought nutritional yeast had a funky, delicious flavor, to the person who discovered that silken tofu makes an awesome chocolate mousse, and to the person who first realized you could milk nuts—I stand on your collective shoulders.

ABOUT THE AUTHOR

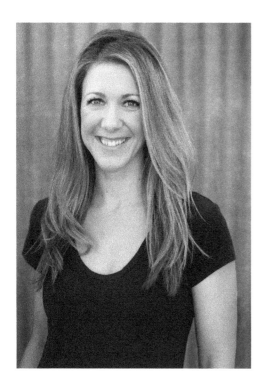

Pamela Ellgen is the author of more than a dozen books on healthy cooking and fitness and the creator of the food blog SurfGirlEats.com. Her work has also been published on Huffington Post, LIVESTRONG, and Edible, and in *Darling Magazine* and the *Portland Tribune*. She lives in Santa Barbara, California, with her husband and two sons. When she's not in the kitchen, she enjoys surfing, building sand castles, and exploring the local farmers' market.

CPSIA information can be obtained
at www.ICGtesting.com
Printed in the USA
ŁVHW07s2111200218
567284LV00009B/21/P

9 781939 754585